Occupational Therapy Across Cultural Boundaries: Theory, Practice and Professional Development

Occupational Therapy Across Cultural Boundaries: Theory, Practice and Professional Development

Susan Cook Merrill
Editor

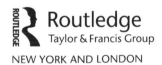

Routledge
Taylor & Francis Group

NEW YORK AND LONDON

First Published by 1992
The Haworth Press, Inc., 10 Alice Street, Binghamton, NY 13904-1580

Published 2010 by Routledge
711 Third Avenue, New York, NY 10017
2 Park Square, Milton Park, Abingdon, Oxfordshire OX14 4RN

First issued in paperback 2016

Routledge is an imprint of the Taylor and Francis Group, an informa business

Occupational Therapy Across Cultural Boundaries: Theory, Practice and Professional Development has also been published as *Occupational Therapy in Health Care*, Volume 8, Number 1 1992.

Library of Congress Cataloging-in-Publication Data

Occupational therapy across cultural boundaries: theory, practice, and professional development/ Susan Cook Merrill, editor.
    p. cm.
    "Has also been published as Occupational therapy in health care, volume 8, number 1" – T.p. verso.
    Includes bibliographical references.
    ISBN 1-56024-223-X (alk. paper)
    1. Occupational therapy. 2. Transcultural medical care. I. Merrill, Susan Cook.
RM735.0298 1992
615.8'515 – dc20   92-36744
                                                    CIP

ISBN 13: 978-1-138-97738-9 (pbk)
ISBN 13: 978-1-56024-223-9 (hbk)

Publisher's Note
The publisher has gone to great lengths to ensure the quality of this reprint but points out that some imperfections in the original may be apparent.

Occupational Therapy Across Cultural Boundaries: Theory, Practice and Professional Development

Occupational Therapy
Across Cultural Boundaries:
Theory, Practice
and Professional Development

CONTENTS

ABOUT THE EDITOR

Susan Cook Merrill, MA, OTR/L, is a part-time instructor in the Department of Occupational Therapy at the University of New Hampshire. She has worked in virtually all domains of physical dysfunction with patients of all ages, both in and out of hospitals, and has held several staff positions, as well as consulting and supervisory positions in occupational therapy programs. She has been a member of the American Occupational Therapy Association since 1974, and was the recipient of two research grants from Thomas Jefferson University, Philadelphia, Pennsylvania. In addition to publishing a number of articles, she edited the book *Environment: Implications for Occupational Therapy Practice: A Sensory Integrative Perspective*, and co-authored the book *Outcomes of Stroke Rehabilitation: Research Resources and Implications for Occupational Therapy*.

Occupational Therapy Across Cultural Boundaries: Theory, Practice and Professional Development

Preface

This issue of *Occupational Therapy in Health Care* examines the concept of culture from the unique perspective of individual occupational therapists who have worked in environments very different from their own. The definition of *culture* is an issue long debated by anthropologists (White, 1959). One definition which seems most relevant for occupational therapists is that culture is the body of shared and learned assumptions, beliefs, symbols and ways of behaving which characterize a human society (Harrison and Ritenbaugh, 1981; Hoebel, 1971). Culture is the knowledge that we acquire as members of a human group which enables us to make sense of our surroundings, both animate and inanimate, and to behave in ways which are understandable to those around us. Culture consists of standards we use to decide what is, what is possible, how we feel about it, what we can do about it, and how to go about doing it (Goodenough, 1963).

Culture is considered the major human adaptation (Hoebel, 1971). It provides the means through which we come to terms with the environment and with each other. Since it is the aspect of human behavior which is based on learning, thought and the use of symbols, culture defines the importance of certain objects, how they will be used, what people will do and how they will do it. Our ability to adapt to recurrent situations by remembering and analyzing the past and our ability to adjust our behavior as new situations confront us are both rooted in our ability to create and maintain culture (Montagu & Matson, 1979).

Since human behavior, like that of all living creatures, derives from our biological capacities, anthropologists believe that culture has its basis in our brain structure (Alland, 1980; Hoebel, 1971). These mechanisms determine how and what we learn and how we organize that information. If these mechanisms create the *potential* for learning, the *actual* learning depends on our experiences in the

xiii

world. Culture, therefore, is the result of biological capacities which enable humans to adapt to the physical and social world in a unique way. These biological capacities are set in motion by human interaction with the animate and inanimate environment.

This issue of *Occupational Therapy in Health Care* describes the experiences of occupational therapists who have crossed cultural boundaries both in professional activities and in day-to-day living. These authors have had the opportunity to practice in settings very different from those they had encountered previously. Unlike living and practicing in one's own culture, these experiences are more demanding of therapists' personal and professional skills. Instead of relying on comfortable, pre-existing cultural maps (Ritenbaugh, 1982), each of these authors was forced to reassess and reconstruct basic assumptions of both personal and professional life.

To help them focus on the unique aspects of their experiences, the authors were given a series of questions which can be found at the end of this introduction. As can be seen, the nature of these questions and the experiences themselves have resulted in articles which are different in tone from articles typically encountered in our professional literature. While each article reflects the author's unique blending of idiosyncratic ideas and internalization of our diverse "American" culture, when taken together, the articles illuminate several well-accepted characteristics of the concept of culture.

First, culture cannot always be verbalized by the members of the group (Hall, 1982). When someone breaks a cultural rule, even if we are not completely aware of it, we are uncomfortable because interpretation and understanding of the individual's behavior becomes difficult. Wilson-Braun, for example, portrays well the conflict she felt when she encountered the different value placed on time and on planning by the Ecuadorean therapists with whom she worked. Fudge, too, in recounting her experiences in Guatemala, provides valuable insight into the emotional upheaval that can result from encountering different cultural values placed on setting and attaining goals with patients.

A second characteristic of culture is that, even though much of the knowledge is not conscious, the standards can be made explicit; they can be learned and studied (Spradley & McCurdy, 1972). This makes cross-cultural communication possible. Slavik, in her article on teaching sensory integration to therapists in Finland, provides excellent guidelines for ensuring effective communication across language and cultural boundaries. Evans' thought-provoking article on schizophrenia in Zanzibar demonstrates how essential understanding cultural explanations of phenomena can be to implementing theory-based practice.

Another characteristic of culture is that the symbolic nature of objects, and therefore how they are used, is defined by an interaction between the culture and the environment (Montagu & Matson, 1979). Miller, for example, in her important work in Cambodia, found that the children there did not have the background experiences with objects to enable them to complete developmental assessment using tests standardized in the United States. Understanding the turmoil and trauma these children have experienced in their young lives led Miller to observe the interaction and movement skills of each child in a very different way than she had expected. Markewitz, in her interesting article on her fieldwork experience in Alaska, describes how the natural resources, the weather and the seasons directly influence the value people living in Sitka place on time and also have a direct relationship to valued activities in everyday life. She further discusses how the isolation of therapists in Alaska led her to develop skills for networking that she might not have needed in another environment.

And finally, there are aspects of the human spirit that appear to transcend cultural boundaries (Montagu, 1950). Both Wilson-Braun and Fudge demonstrate the universality of the needs of people with disabilities. They also provide us with excellent illustrations of the relevance of occupational therapy skills to other cultures. Miller, in working with Cambodian children rediscovered the intrinsic joy that comes when a child plays with a ball or balloon; a joy that has no cultural boundaries.

Each of these articles has much more to offer than the brief points highlighted above. Of keen interest to the reader will be each author's discussion of the effect the experiences have had on her, both professionally and personally. Each article is an eloquent statement of how experiencing other cultures creates the opportunity for personal growth. It is the opinion of the authors and the editor that we have much to learn from sharing these experiences.

Several of the contributors to this volume are first-time authors and it has been rewarding to work with them. My thanks to all the authors for their willingness to contribute to our literature despite the long hours of writing and revision. I am also grateful to the members of the Editorial Board who, under arduous time limits, reviewed these articles and provided thoughtful and thorough comments to the authors.

Susan Cook Merrill, MA, OTR/L

QUESTIONS FOR AUTHORS

1. Explain how and why you happened to become involved in the situation you are writing about.

2. What information about the socio-political-economics and health care needs of the situation are relevant?

3. What background information about you (e.g., years of practice, practice settings in the United States prior to your trip) is relevant?

4. What were your expectations of the situation and of your role before you got there?

5. Describe occupational therapy practice: this should be thick description to give the reader a real feeling for your experiences, for example: living and working environments, the clients/patients, your role as an OT, the hours you worked, the number of people you treated in a day, how you modified both theory and practice from what you do/did in the United States.

6. What were positive and negative aspects of your experience? How did this experience change you in both positive and negative ways?

7. What did it feel like to return to living and practicing in an environment more familiar to you?

8. How has your practice changed as a result of this experience — in evaluation, treatment, frames of reference? What do you do differently now that you think is directly related to your experience?

REFERENCES

Alland, A. (1980). *To be human. An introduction to anthropology*. New York: John Wiley & Sons, Inc.

Goodenough, W.H. (1963). *Cooperation in change*. New York: Russell Sage Foundation.

Hall, E.T. (1982). *The hidden dimension*. Garden City, NY: Anchor Books.

Harrison G.G. & Ritenbaugh, C. (1981). Anthropology and nutrition: A perspective on two scientific subcultures. *Federation Proceedings, 40* 2595-2600.

Hoebel, E.A. (1971). The nature of culture. In H.L. Shapiro (Ed.), *Man, culture and society*. (pp. 208-222). London: Oxford University Press.

Montagu, A. (1950). *On being human*. New York: Henry Schuman.

Montagu, A. & Matson, F. (1979). *The human connection*. New York: McGraw-Hill Book Company.

Ritenbaugh, C. (1982). New approaches to old problems: Interactions of culture and nutrition. In N.J. Chrisman & T.W. Maretzki (Eds.), *Clinically applied anthropology. Anthropologists in health science settings*. (pp. 141-178). Boston: D. Reidel Publishing Company.

Spradley, J.P. & McCurdy, D.W. (1972). *The cultural experience. Ethnography in complex society*. Chicago: Science Research Associates, Inc.

White, L.A. (1959). The concept of culture. In A. Montagu (Ed.), *Culture and the evolution of man*. (pp. 38-64). New York: Oxford University Press.

An Occupational Therapy Experience in Ecuador

Carol E. Wilson-Braun, MA, OTR/L

SUMMARY. This paper describes the experiences of the author, her husband and a physical therapist who travelled to Ecuador in 1989 for three months to volunteer in their professions. It highlights aspects of health care in that country and of occupational therapy education and practice. It focuses on their teaching experiences in various settings and on their participation in the development of a daily living skills program for the disabled.

My husband Jeff and I are Occupational Therapists, and have worked in the Boston area in physical rehabilitation settings for almost seven and six years, respectively. For a long time, we had wanted to volunteer abroad, especially in the area of occupational therapy, if possible. We did not feel ready to commit to a full two years, as the Peace Corps requires, but were more comfortable with an experience of three month's duration.

We preferred Latin America since we both speak intermediate levels of Spanish and had visited several countries there previously. I had relatives in Ecuador who had extended invitations for family to visit, and who told us they knew of some volunteer opportunities, so our decision was made! After obtaining leaves of absence from our workplaces in March of 1989, we travelled to Ecuador, accompanied by Ellen Rohan, a physical therapist and friend of ours.

We worked completely independently of any organization, and

Carol E. Wilson-Braun is a Registered Occupational Therapist and Resource Clinician at Braintree Hospital, 250 Pond St., Braintree, MA 02184. Her co-travellers were her husband Jeff Wilson-Braun, OTR/L, who works at Spaulding Rehabilitation Hospital in Boston, MA, and Ellen Rohan, PT, who works at New England Rehabilitation Hospital in Woburn, MA.

1

were able to establish connections with various schools and institutions through our relatives and their friends. We went with the expectation of doing direct care in hospitals and clinics, working alongside Ecuadorean occupational therapists, and being able to observe in different settings. This was only one of many expectations that was modified during our travels.

Early in our stay, we were taken on a tour of several public and private hospitals in Quito, the capital of Ecuador, by a physical therapist friend of my family's who acted as our liaison. As we talked about where we could fit in, we realized that what was wanted of us was not direct patient care but teaching. We were unprepared to discover that we were considered experts, coming from the United States, and everyone wanted us to teach courses and lead workshops! At that time, Jeff had five years and I four years experience (Ellen had three years) and did not consider ourselves experts by any stretch of the imagination. Although it made us uncomfortable and a bit nervous, we decided we would teach what we could. The challenge for us was to keep ourselves open and flexible, both to what therapists wanted from us and to the lifestyle of Ecuador.

ECUADOR
AND ITS HEALTH CARE SYSTEM

Ecuador is a small mountainous country that straddles the equator in South America. Quito, where we spent most of our time, is a sprawling city situated between mountains (actually an extinct volcano crater) about 9000 feet above sea level. Its population is currently about a million people and includes a large percentage of indigenous people, who are descended from the Incas. In recent years, the city has mushroomed with poor people from the rural parts of the country who have come looking for jobs and a better standard of living. There are not enough jobs and living is difficult. The life expectancy is 60 years and the literacy rate is 74%. The per capita income is $1,050 and one half of Ecuador's population is made up of subsistence farmers (National Geographic Society, 1981).

The most frequently encountered general medical problems in

Ecuador are parasites, tuberculosis, alcoholism, diarrhea and malnutrition (Braun, 1989). The diagnoses we saw most frequently were orthopedic (fractures and spinal cord injuries from falls, motor vehicle accidents or other trauma), burns, and neurological (either peripheral nerve injuries or cerebrovascular accidents).

We visited a number of hospitals in Quito, representing the four kinds of health care systems in Ecuador: government or "poor people's" hospitals, social security hospitals and military hospitals (also government run) and private hospitals. In general, the government hospitals were older with more patients on a ward, but they offered free care, and so were what most people could afford. The private hospitals were on the other end of the continuum, being newer, with state-of-the-art technology and semi-private rooms.

The Suarez Hospital was a 120-bed government hospital for poor people. It employed two occupational therapists, four physical therapists and one speech therapist who worked primarily with outpatients, less with inpatients. They often used an interdisciplinary team approach, especially with pediatric patients. In the occupational therapy room, there were various pegs, cones and equipment for upper extremity strengthening and coordination.

The Social Security Hospital was only for people in the social security system, not even their families. There was one occupational therapist and several physical therapists. The occupational therapist was also a general practitioner who practiced occupational therapy in the morning and medicine in the afternoon! The two occupational therapy rooms contained a kiln, drill, copper tooling and other crafts (when the materials are available), a small ADL corner, two pottery wheels, standing tables and a skateboard platform. The rooms seemed average in size for occupational therapy clinics, and we were surprised by how much equipment they did have, though it might be considered sparse by some of our standards. Much of the equipment was handmade, such as ADL boards and fine motor coordination boards with various latches and switches. The occupational therapist would typically see 40 patients in a six hour period.

The military hospital was a 400-bed hospital for members of the military and their families. The occupational therapists there each saw 20 to 25 patients each shift. Diagnoses included hemiplegia, arthritis and upper extremity problems. Activities focused largely on fine and gross motor coordination using looms, macrame, crocheting, ceramics, ADL boards and small blocks.

Finally, the Metropolitan Hospital was a private two-year-old 120-bed hospital for wealthy people who could pay independently. It offered physical therapy only, which had rooms well set up with mats, mirrors, bolsters, parallel bars, and included a variety of sophisticated instruments such as for cardiac rehabilitation.

OCCUPATIONAL THERAPY IN ECUADOR

There are four occupational therapy schools in Ecuador, each with its own curriculum and final exam. At this time there is no standard curriculum for occupational therapy nor a national exam. All are three year schools and students are graduated with the title of medical technician in occupational therapy. The program includes practical experience for half of the second and third years, with students spending only one month at a time at each clinic site. We looked at the curriculum and found it similar to what one would find in the United States: First year—history of occupational therapy, terminology, multi-disciplinary rehabilitation teams, basic principles of treatment (evaluation and treatment planning), physiology; second year—practicals in the mornings, and in the afternoons, classes such as treatment planning, range of motion and resistive exercises, facilitation and inhibition techniques, O.T. and mental health, ADL's, and in the third year—practicals in the mornings and classes such as neuromuscular techniques (including Bobath, Rood, Brunnstrom and Fuchs), arthritis, amputations, and splinting and orthotics in the afternoons.

There are no formal occupational therapy organizations at any level although some students and therapists are trying to start an association in Ecuador. A group of people was submitting a paper last year to the Ministry of Health, with the hope of starting a national association, and then joining the Latin American Association of Occupational Therapy and then the World Federation of Occupational Therapy. At the present, the occupational therapists in Ecuador feel cut off from many resources because of their isolation from therapy associations in the United States and other countries. Those therapists we met expressed great enthusiasm for their profession and a strong desire for communication with occupational therapists in the United States.

There is a shortage of jobs for occupational therapists in Ecuador, especially in the cities, so there is great competition for jobs. This appears to have the unfortunate effect of decreasing networking among therapists. For example, one therapist showed us an evaluation she had developed but asked us not to share it with any other therapists.

From what we observed, the emphasis of occupational therapy appears to be on crafts, upper extremity strengthening and coordination, and Daily Living skills. The general response when we did mat work or trunk and balance work (such as with NDT/Bobath techniques) was that we were doing physical therapy! There seems to be very little if any overlap with physical therapy (again perhaps due to the high level of competition. Physical therapists, as well as doctors, defend their turf fiercely because of the lack of jobs). Many hospitals and clinics are poorly funded and lack materials. In one clinic we visited, the occupational therapist sent his patients out to the store to buy their own materials. Therapists generally see 20 to 30 patients a day. Therapists usually treat several patients simultaneously. Individual therapy is brief, 15 minute sessions. The salary for one therapist we met was 36,000 sucres per month, which is about $72. However, in relation to the economy in Ecuador and the range of salaries, according to people we met, this was not too different from our salaries at home.

The referral process for both outpatients and inpatients appeared to be similar to the referral system we know in the United States; through a physician. However, referrals for therapy often seemed to come much later than in the United States, with most of the patients we observed seen as outpatients rather than inpatients. One young man had just been referred for therapy three months after a severe burn to one of his arms. He had medical care including grafts, which were healing well, but he had severe contractures of his fingers, wrist and elbow, so any prognosis of improvement was guarded at that point. We started making a dynamic splint and range of motion exercise program for him but he stopped coming in. We were disappointed at the lost opportunity to help him. The therapists were not able to reach him before we left the area. The therapists speculated that because he lived with his mother he probably was not able to support himself and so therapy was not relevant to him.

We saw a woman who had fallen five months earlier and fractured both elbows and had been casted from her hands up past her elbows. Now her elbows were contracted at 90° and she had also lost a lot of range of her shoulders, wrists and fingers. Apparently she had not exercised her shoulders and hands while her elbows were immobilized. We were able to help her obtain some increased range after a short session of prolonged stretch and contract/relax techniques. We would have liked to teach the therapists some joint mobilization techniques but since our time with those therapists was limited, we did not want to leave them with a little knowledge that might do more harm than good.

On another occasion, we were invited up to a ward by some nurses who wanted to learn more about positioning and transfers for a young man with quadriplegia. We arranged for his mother to be there as well, emphasizing to the nurses and therapists the importance of family teaching. His injury had been four years earlier and his visits to the hospital were for medical management of respiratory and skin problems. Otherwise he would sit at home all day in a wheelchair, with his mother carrying him to bed at night. He was in the hospital now with a large decubitus. We demonstrated to the mother and nurses about bed positioning and the importance of changing his position every two to three hours instead of letting him lie all night or sit all day in his chair. We demonstrated how to help him achieve comfortable positions in supine, prone and sidelying using pillows, whereas before, he had been comfortable only in prone and supine. Again, we felt acutely the need to provide more training, but time did not allow us to discuss either range of motion exercises or self-feeding techniques. The therapists that worked at that hospital in Ambato seemed to work primarily with outpatients. We were aware of only a couple of inpatient referrals during the time we were there.

In all but one of the clinics we visited, we saw no evidence of formal evaluations. The therapists were apparently not accustomed to re-evaluating status (for example, joint range of motion), so monitoring progress and effectiveness of treatment was more difficult. As a result, patients could be kept on treatment for months even if little progress was made. It seemed as though patients' length of stay was limited by their ability to pay (if private) and not by the external pressures of third party payors. There was some paperwork involved, but very little compared to what we are used to in the United States. The absence of third party payors in the health care system seemed to be the reason behind the differences in paperwork and general accountability.

TEACHING EXPERIENCES

We had the opportunity to teach on three separate occasions: a two-day course at the private Metropolitan Hospital for occupational and physical therapists in the Quito area, a one-week course at a hospital in the nearby city of Ambato for occupational and physical therapists, nurses and some physicians, and a one-week course for occupational and physical therapy students at the Central University in Quito.

The Physical Therapy Association was sponsoring a stroke conference at the Metropolitan Hospital. When the planning committee learned that we were in the area, they asked if we would consider teaching part of the conference. We agreed to teach one half day of the two-day conference. As the time drew near for the conference, it became apparent to us that it was not taking shape at all, as no other speakers had been asked. In the United States, we are used to conferences which are planned many months in advance. Not so in Ecuador! Time is perceived and used differently there; slower paced and less rigid. The week before the conference, we learned that we *were* the conference! This was quite a surprise to us. We had no obligation nor were we prepared to present an entire conference, and we considered cancelling. But since we had already put a lot of work into it, we felt we should carry through on our part, and so decided to go ahead and present two half days. We were learning how important it was to be flexible!

The content was entirely left up to us. We arranged for an interpreter and for a wheelchair and plinth as props. We were quite amazed on the first morning to have an audience of 100 people! Our course content covered such topics as body mechanics, transfers, orthopedic exercises and stretching techniques, bed and wheelchair positioning, abnormal tone, skin care, exercises and ambulation, and treating the hemiplegic upper and lower extremities. It sounds very ambitious, but we covered only the very basics. We were advised by the physical therapy liaison with whom we worked to keep the content of what we taught basic and practical. She told us that students get a lot of theory in school but not a lot of practical application. They sit through many lectures but do not get much hands-on experience (Erickson, 1989). In this course, as well as all the others we organized during our stay, we emphasized physical management of patients. We sought to complement the therapy we saw being done in clinics that focused on upper extremity strengthening and coordination and crafts.

In Ambato, we again taught a basic course focusing on orthopedic and neurological dysfunction, positioning and treatment techniques. We were able to have a local physical therapist and a physician interpret for us.

Jeff and I were asked to teach a course during our stay at the occupational therapy school at the Central University. We persuaded the president of the school that one week would be fine for us, instead of a month, and asked him what they would like taught, what would fit into their course schedule. With a politeness we encountered over and over, he insisted that anything we wanted to teach would be fine. So much for direction. Upon the advice of our physical therapist liaison in Quito, we made the content basic and practical. As the week approached, we learned that we would be teaching the third year class of physical therapy students as well as the third year class of occupational therapy students, in effect tripling the class from 20 to 60. Also, the class would be held at a nearby government hospital instead of the school.

The teaching experiences provided us with a valuable lesson: we learned to just "hang loose," for events often proceeded at what we considered a very relaxed pace. For example, the first day of the University course, we arrived at the rehab unit promptly at 1:15 p.m. to meet our translator and set up for the 2 p.m. class. At 1:45 p.m. she arrived, closely followed by the director of the school to greet us. We were informed that the class would take place either right there in the hallway or in the outpatient clinic. We asked what would happen to patients if we held class in the clinic and were told that all the afternoon patients would be cancelled! We decided to use the hallway, but found that it was dim, crowded and noisy. There was a loudspeaker right above us. We asked the students if they wanted to switch to the clinic the next day and they agreed. We discovered that the patients' appointments had been cancelled anyway because the therapists were attending the class! The clinic was still crowded and many students stood the entire three hours, but there were plinths and a wider space.

Because of the third party reimbursement system and health care crisis in the United States, we would never consider cancelling patient treatment for an entire afternoon for a course. We would shift our schedules around so that some therapists could go and their caseloads be covered, or we would treat in a different location so the course could take place and we could still continue treating. In Ecuador, our being there pre-empted patient care. We felt respected and honored as guests, but still the whole situation seemed very "last minute" to us.

Our content for this course included body mechanics, bed mobility and transfers (so students could learn and practice the movements), assessment and treatment of tone in the upper extremity, Daily Living Skills, cognition and perception. We also covered management of some orthopedic and neuromuscular issues because we had seen patients with contractures in the clinics.

For the last day, we had asked for three volunteer patients so we could demonstrate treatment techniques used with spastic and flaccid hemiplegia and a person with orthopedic contractures. The two patients that came in were more challenging than we anticipated; they were at the extreme ends of the continuum between spastic and flaccid. We had planned to demonstrate facilitation and inhibition techniques, but for the former patient, serial casting would have been more appropriate, and for the latter, a sling or just positioning was all we could do. We explained this to the students and utilized the opportunity to discuss serial casting and the importance of positioning and slings. We demonstrated on each other various facilitation and inhibition techniques.

We encountered another challenge when teaching transfer techniques. In the United States, we are used to being able to vary bed heights for smooth and safe squat-pivot or sliding board transfers, but what does one do when the bed is three feet high and on non-locking casters, and the wheelchair is old with non-removable arm-rests and footrests? *And* the patient is five feet tall? When we dem-onstrated, our feet touched the floor for a squat-pivot, but a student volunteer was so short, we ended up adapting the squat-pivot as well as teaching a two-person lift!

CASA APA

We became involved with Campamento Nueva Vida, a small ec-umenical group camp situated in the small town of La Merced out-side of Quito, when they decided to start a program for the disabled. Jeff, Ellen and I, and a nurse and a teacher from the United States, along with a doctor and others from Ecuador were charged with developing a short-term daily living skills program for 12 clients. People from around Ecuador with diagnoses such as paraplegia, arthritis, amputations and heart conditions would come for an aver-age of three months for respite and rehabilitation.

Ellen, Jeff and I prepared a week of training for the camp staff. They had no previous experience working with disabled people, so we focused on explaining some of the disabilities they would be seeing, raising consciousness about disabilities through simula-tions, and discussing realistic goals for people with these problems.

The program was housed in a building called House of Love, Peace and Friendship, or Casa APA in Spanish, and contained two six-bed dormitories for men and women, a kitchen, dining room, two bathrooms and two large activity rooms. We were told that Casa APA had been designed as accessible housing. Although doorways were plenty wide we found that the shower stalls had four inch rims and regular showerheads, and there were cabinets with doors under the kitchen counter, among other things. We made rec-ommendations to the director and the head of maintenance for changes as funds were available. They appreciated our input since they had not much experience with individuals with disabilities.

We were also consulted for dimensions and wheelchair accessi-bility when a pila was built outside the house. A pila is a free-standing double basin for washing clothes. The gas and water had not yet been hooked up, nor other things finished when we found out on a Friday that the clients would all be arriving the next day! So much for advanced notice. We had to house them in other buildings on the campground for about a week until Casa APA was ready.

We came to realize that the ideal accessible set-up for us was unrealistic for these people, for even if the house was made fully accessible, people would be returning to their homes which would not be accessible or likely to become so. For example, I interviewed a young woman with paraparesis about her set-up at home. When I asked her about her bathroom (my thoughts being, of course, things like door width and wheelchair accessibility and location of fixtures), she replied that her bathroom was outside the house, down a path, then down some steps to the back yard!

We helped to set up an interview/evaluation procedure and a program, chosen by the director, of sewing, ceramics, crafts and woodworking, to which we added exercises and Daily Living Skills. These activities were chosen to provide leisure outlets for the clients, but also to teach them self-care and homemaking skills and possibly help them learn skills to become wage earners again.

The director of the camp saw the program as providing respite for the clients' families, as well as a chance for people to learn new skills. It was our hope, even though we were involved with this project for a short period of time, that the residents of the house would start assuming control of the running of the house, including planning the menus, ordering food and cooking the meals, making the beds, cleaning the house, doing their laundry and so on. These people, unlike those born with disabilities, had been productive adults until becoming disabled, and so had not been dependent on others for very long. They were used to doing things for themselves.

Sometimes in Ecuador, we were told, disabled people are hidden away, out of sight, and stay in bed all day long. Often, the case is that very few families are able to afford equipment or therapy, so people unable to walk are confined to beds and couches and are completely dependent on their families carrying them or crawling from place to place. If they cannot work, they become a financial burden to their struggling families. Sometimes they are abandoned and left to beg. We also discovered that there is a tendency to infantilize people with disabilities — to make decisions for them and tell them what to do.* All control and choice are taken away. These attitudes toward disabled people make it very hard to work toward the goals we set for the clients in the program. And indeed, as we left, we found the camp management setting rules and schedules for the clients. We wished we could have stayed longer to influence the project further, although it is unclear how much influence we might have had. It would be interesting at this point to see how Ecuadorean therapists who have taken our places have dealt with what we see as the conflicting philosophies of the camp and of occupational therapy. For in therapy, we work toward a person's self-actualization and becoming independently functioning.

CONCLUSION

Our experiences in Ecuador were very rewarding for us. It took time to establish connections and set up courses, so that most of our activity took place during the last of our three months. As our time of departure approached, we felt we were just getting started with what we came to do, but we left with the hope of returning another year to do more teaching and work beside the therapists in the clinics. We did not do as much hands-on work with patients as we had hoped or sharing of knowledge with Ecuadorean therapists. The need communicated to us was for teaching again and again (though ironically, the content was continually left up to us!). This was both puzzling and frustrating to us, because we wanted to augment what they already knew. We wanted to give them something new, but they, in being polite and gracious to us, would not give us specific suggestions, nor did they let us know afterward if they already had learned what we presented. All we could do was present as best we could and hope that it was worthwhile to them. They were always very appreciative.

We realized in retrospect that teaching students and therapists had made a larger impact than if we had just spent our time treating

---

*We never had to deal specifically with the differences in values because we were there such a short time.

patients. We also realized that to be more effective, a stay of at least six months to a year would be preferable.

We were also very fortunate to have relatives in Ecuador through whom we made our connections. Unless therapists wishing to volunteer already have some connections in the country they plan to visit, it is probably a good idea to go with an established group or volunteer organization that has already laid the groundwork.

Our professional exchange was limited by our language skills. We each knew enough Spanish to express ourselves in informal situations, but our lack of fluency kept discussions with therapists at a basic level. For the formal courses and teaching situations, we were fortunate to have the volunteer services of various interpreters. The work pace was relaxed, and we were surprised (if not a little envious) when therapists and other medical professionals would take off half and full days on short notice to attend our conferences.

Upon returning to our respective rehabilitation settings in the Boston area, we were amazed at the wealth of our own society and the richness of resources and equipment available at our hospitals. Providing therapy is easy with modern wheelchairs, sliding boards, a variety of equipment and the luxury of long individual treatment sessions with each patient. We are also fortunate to have the opportunity to attend conferences on any number of topics. It was at times sad and frustrating to see patients who could have benefitted from more timely or sophisticated treatment such as we have, and we felt helpless in being able to make any kind of a difference especially during a short-term visit. But we remember also that there are many people in this country who have no access to the technology of our health care system.

While our treatment techniques have not changed as a result of our experience in Ecuador, we have gained greater perspective and appreciation of the wealth of our health care system in general, as well as an appreciation and respect for the people we met in Ecuador who work without these resources. Our day-to-day professional activities allow us to lose perspective on our situation, never having experienced anything very different. Our way of life in this country is privileged beyond what most of the world can dream of. Our own lives have been greatly enriched by the challenges of our time in Ecuador.

REFERENCES

Braun, Helen. (1989). Peace Corps Nurse in Quito, Ecuador. Personal communication.

Erickson, Sheryl. (1989). Physical Therapist in Quito, Ecuador. Personal communication.

National Geographic Society. (1981). National Geographic Atlas of the World, (5th ed.). Washington, D.C.

A Perspective on Consulting in Guatemala

Sara Fudge, MHS, OTR/L

SUMMARY. Attempting to offer short-term help in a center for disabled, delayed and nutritionally deprived children in Antigua Guatemala was quite a learning experience. Good intentions and conventional Northern approaches often collided with reality, providing the author with perhaps as many learning experiences as she was able to provide to the center.

My friend Judith is a story teller and adventurer. She weaves the most incredible stories from her life. Back in our twenties, when everyone else was meditating or doing yoga, her spiritual practice was to hitchhike. Judith would get out on the highway, say a prayer and stick out her thumb. When someone stopped to offer her a ride, she would try to read their energy to see if it was safe. She never took a ride she did not feel comfortable with. And nothing bad ever happened. She did, however, have the most incredible stories to tell. I have never tired of listening to them. Judith is also a Montessori teacher who dearly loves children. When she announced to her friends that she was taking a leave of absence from her teaching job to go work in some children's center in Guatemala, we were not too surprised. Back for Christmas the next year, her stories spun a web that I could not resist. That March, I was off to Guatemala for a visit.

I have never been farther from the United States than Canada or Mexico. I knew I was in for a culture shock, but I could not fathom the nature of what might happen. Arriving in the airport in Guate-

Sara Fudge is clinical instructor at the University of Puget Sound and is in private practice. Her address is: 11011 32nd Ave. E., Seattle, WA 98112.

15

mala City, flanked by soldiers holding machine guns, remembering the stories of kidnap and murder in this country, hearing only Spanish, I became fearful of making a wrong move. Not knowing Spanish, my brain responded to a foreign language with the only alternative I had. I started thinking and responding in broken French. How embarrassing.

Judith and I soon turned my lack of Spanish to our advantage. When it was best to be the ignorant gringa, as when men were trying to pick us up, I would speak for us; "no comprende" I would say, looking puzzled. She was gaining fluency and became our spokeswoman when it was to our advantage to know Spanish. Thus, at the market, she would bargain hard, while I would get "bored" and walk away, panicking the market sellers into coming down on their prices.

We did not feel bad about driving hard bargains because Judith was living on Guatemalan wages, but being charged gringo prices. No matter how hard she bargained, she never did get local prices, and found it less expensive to hire a Mayan woman to shop for her groceries and do her laundry too, rather than to pay the prices she could get herself. Judith taught English to the rich Guatemalan kids to support herself. She then volunteered at the Obras Socialies del Hermano Pedro, otherwise known as the Casa. The Casa was an old hospital turned residential center for a variety of disabled children and adults in the heart of the old capital of Antigua. Antigua is earthquake prone and the capital eventually moved down onto a more stable plain, leaving many magnificent old Spanish structures in partial ruin to grace the city with mystery. The hospital was a newer ruin which the city gave to Friar Guillermo Bonillo Carvajal, a Franciscan friar from Costa Rica, in the 1980s. The Friar had been taking in physically handicapped children and caring for them in a scattering of homes around the city.

There is no State help for disabled people in Guatemala. Most families are very poor, and all members of the family are needed to earn a living. According to the Nutritional Institute for Central America and Panama, Guatemalans need $10.40 a day to feed an average family. The minimum wage was $3.20 a day and unemployment ran at 52 per cent in 1986 (Acker, 1986). When a child is unable to contribute to the family, needs constant supervision or has major medical needs, the strain on the family is intolerable. If the child cannot tend the kitchen, make craft items, or beg, the family often cannot subsidize his or her existence in the home. The Friar provided a humane alternative. When Judith arrived at the Casa, she found a very clean, gentle place where the children had three meals a day, were bathed regularly, had clean clothes and routine medical care.

Judith befriended a ward of teenage boys who were all wheel chair-bound with such conditions as cerebral palsy, spina bifida and polio. These boys were curious and bored. She began a program of reading, writing, and math, translating English curriculum into Spanish. When I came, I found myself immediately eyeing their positions in the wheelchairs and their patterns of movement. So ingrained was my neurodevelopmental training as an occupational therapist, that I soon had several of the boys out of their wheelchairs. I moved them around on the floor, stretching tight muscles, facilitating balance reactions, trying to stimulate normal movement patterns. I had the same reaction on the ward for girls with mental retardation. This time from a sensory integration and human occupation perspective I was assessing their environment, looking for activities that would stimulate their senses, teach them problem solving skills, help them learn functional skills. Having no materials at hand, I simply picked up the girls, swinging them around, playing little give and take social interaction games with them. Nursing and domestic care workers walked by me, grinning, but remained very adult in their behavior. The children became mine, and I became intensely interested in trying to find ways to make their lives meaningful (Photo 1).

The purpose of my trip was to visit Judith and see the country with someone who could take me beyond the tourist hangouts. But as we traveled around, I found myself checking out the markets and stores trying to assess what indigenous items could be used to act as therapeutic material. While there were no toys or simple learning games in the markets, many items that could be used in sensory integration activities were to be found. I was constantly pointing these things out to Judith and explaining to her how hammocks and tire swings and interesting textures could stimulate and enhance the functioning of these children. As we traveled about, I began lectur-

PHOTO 1. The author cleans out a tightly fisted hand.

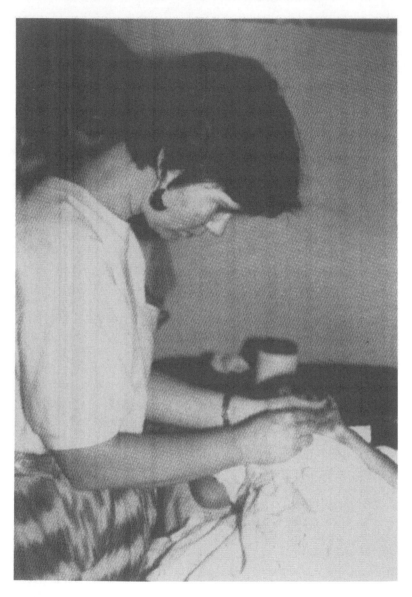

ing her on muscle tone problems and sensory stimulation techniques.

One day, while traveling by boat across Lake Atitlan, we were temporarily stranded by some unscrupulous boatmen, who took our money and delivered us to a remote pier of a Mayan village. The village was in rebel territory and the people spoke an obscure Mayan tongue. Spanish was a second language for them, too. Nervous, we decided to stay on the beach right by the dock and wait for a boat which might or might not come. The lecture of the day was on the tactile system and we decided it might provide a good distraction. For some reason, I felt compelled to explain touch from an evolutionary perspective and began informing Judith about the invertebrate nervous system. Using sticks and stones, the brain slowly evolved from neural tube to the complex folds of the great apes' cerebrum. All the while, the children of the village had gathered around and were watching the lesson intently. Soon the village cripple had inched over too, scooting along on his bottom, his atrophied legs trailing behind, hands extended for spare change. As my audience grew, I began to speak to them, too. They, in turn, would nod knowingly back at me. My lecture on neurology continued in English until the next boat arrived and took us back to touristdom.

The Casa had a physical therapy department. It was run by a foreign missionary who had taught herself physical therapy techniques using a book. While I admired her assessment that therapy was needed, I was very opinionated about the antiquated techniques being used. Some practices, like standing kids in standing frames without aligning their feet, so that they stood on severely pronated ankle bones quite alarmed me. Patiently, I made appointments and surprise visits trying to gain an audience with this woman and offer her my "wonderful" expertise. The talk never occurred. I left Guatemala feeling like two systems of therapy had been put in place at the Casa, neither one run by a trained therapist. Emotionally, I felt invested in how the children were being cared for and I worried about what would happen next.

Judith came back the next summer with tales of a new nutritional recovery program for infants that had started at the Casa. She was very excited about the effects she had seen of her stimulation program upon the recovering infant's ability to gain weight and develop interaction skills. Immediately we fell into a new round of lectures on infant development. I felt very strongly that she should be assessing the babies with standardized tools. The easiest one for me to get for her and teach her to use was the one I used, the Peabody Fine and Gross Motor Assessment (Folio and Fewell, 1983). Judith headed south that summer bearing boxes of toys and the Peabody. I thought it was relatively culture free, but found out later that it was not.

At Christmas Judith was back, full of technical questions. I was pleased at the level of sophistication she had. While Judith worked to raise money to continue the program, we plotted the growth of her program. Judith wanted to develop a therapy room and to begin to involve Guatemalans in the work. She spoke of the need for people in their own culture to take on the responsibility and vision of what happens in programs like hers. Too often it becomes easy to fall back on the help of foreigners, to become passive and see one's self as a victim of circumstances in which you are helpless.

From an outsider's perspective, the culture of Guatemala can sometimes feel like one big dysfunctional family full of abusers, victims and rescuers. Politics in Guatemala have cycles of intense internal warfare followed by more subdued intimidation. The most recent cycle of violence started in 1978, when General Garcia initiated a period of violence and terror in which eight thousand people died in four years. In 1982, General Rios Montt continued the reign of terror through a "bullets or beans" program. "If you are with us, we'll feed you; if not we'll shoot you," was how one army officer put it (Acker, 1986). Four thousand more died in 1982 alone (Acker, 1986). Many villages in Northern Guatemala were destroyed. Today the New York Times estimates the number of street children in Guatemala City at 10,000 (NYT Magazine, 1.6.91). Amnesty International feels that many of the older children were displaced by the army counter-insurgency campaigns of General Montt. Children and the workers trying to help them, continue to face harassment, threats, attacks, beatings, torture and apparent extrajudicial executions by Guatemala City Police (Amnesty International, 1990). In such a place, teaching people how to effectively help improve conditions for the less fortunate, especially teaching problem solving skills that utilize nearby resources, becomes a political act.

As Judith and I talked over the program, I found myself teaching her more sophisticated techniques. Knowing she would be sharing these with a variety of people, I began to feel it was essential I make a second trip to Guatemala to insure that what I had shared with her was being interpreted correctly. I also felt my heart pulled to go back and help. I decided that this trip would be clearly for the purpose of training and assisting in the program.

Judith suggested two books, *Helping Health Workers Learn* and *Disabled Village Children*, both by David Werner and published by the Hesperian Foundation. I read both eagerly, envisioning how I would spend time listening, observing, finding ways that I could start from the beginning to give the workers at the Casa the information that they thought was most important. I would not impose my values on them. I would serve these people and help them develop the program they wanted, thus empowering them and also ensuring that what was set up would continue because it was their vision, not mine.

When I returned to the Casa, there were many changes. The missionary working in the physical therapy department was gone, replaced by a young Guatemalan man, Oscar, who had been trained as a physical therapist in Costa Rica. An education program complete with classrooms and ten teachers had been added. The new nutritional recovery program for infants and toddlers was in place. A room in the nutritional recovery area had been given over to Judith and she had turned it into a first-rate therapy room; one that most therapists would have been delighted to work in.

Over chocolate, Judith had requested from the States, we planned for the training programs. Four groups of staff had been identified as needing or wanting training: the caretakers or nineras of the infant nutritional recovery program, the education staff, the physical therapy staff, and the nineras that took care of the most severely involved kids. We set up schedules with all of them and began the next day.

My first session with the nutritional recovery nineras was quite an experience. With Judith translating, I began by asking the women to tell me about their center. That question alone was enough to set off a whole new domain of cultural understanding. It seems that no one asks the nineras things, especially to explain what they do. It also seems that in Central American culture, teachers lecture, often by rote, writing things on the blackboard, and students copy things down. No discussion, no questions. They were very hesitant to start talking. So we brought in a child and I began to ask about the child. First came data; Julio is four years old, weighed 22 pounds when he came, now he weighs 25, an eight percent gain in three weeks. As Julio sat there beaming at the attention, the ninras relaxed and began chattering about his personality and what he did and did not know. The atmosphere changed to one of sharing among friends and within that context, we began to problem solve what to do about Julio's poor development.

Julio had kwashiorkor, a prolonged protein deficiency disease in which the body is forced to consume its own muscle tissue. This typically happens as the child is weaned off the breast onto starchy foods. The child may look alright due to edema, but if one looks closely, one notes flaky skin, thinning and discoloration of hair, emaciated muscles, enlarged belly, and apathy (Merck Manual, 1987). The staff described to me how Julio had come to them irritable, withdrawn and not wanting to be touched. They said this was typical of the children when they came in. Julio would come to the therapy room and sit in the tire swing and watch the other children, never smiling (Photo 2).

The clinical picture of Julio suggested tactile defensiveness to me, with possible gravitational insecurity and motor planning problems. If what the nineras were telling me was true, the sensory integrative status of children with kwashiorkor might be impaired. Since I had no comparison group of children who had not been therapeutically handled, I do not know whether the poor response to sensory input would have resolved in time as the nutritional status of the children improved.

The sensory integration principles I had taught Judith by the lake during the last visit had become an integral part of the children's recovery process. In her room, she had used a tire swing and ham-

PHOTO 2. Judith pushes Julio on the tire swing.

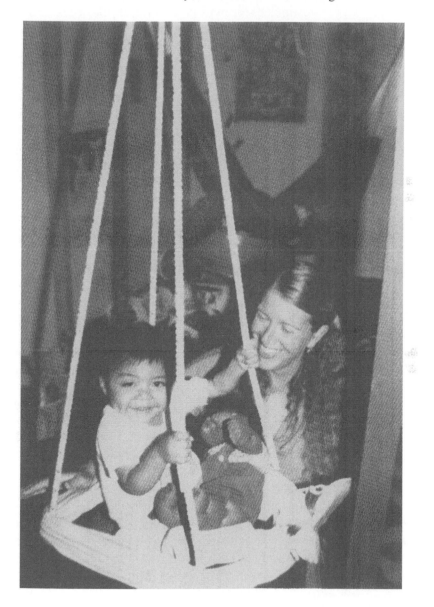

mock (both readily available locally). They turned out to be great ways to provide vestibular stimulation to children too weak to seek it in other ways. The children also gain passive tactile stimulation with firm pressure over large surfaces of their bodies at a time when they are too sensitive to tolerate the seemingly random and spontaneous touch involved in human contact. Firm pressure is often the first approach one uses with desensitizing sensitive skin in children (Oetter, 1984). I was glad to hear that it seemed to help the children with kwashiorkor as their systems recovered in the center. Indeed, Julio was doing very well now, joyously entering into all the activities offered him. Long term prognosis for kwashiorkor includes physical recovery but often mild retardation. It is Judith's hope to provide the kind of environment to lessen the long term retardation and to gain normal muscle and motor development. The first physical goal I saw for Julio was recovery of the abdominals, such a pivotal group of muscles for postural control and equilibrium.

As we came to this point in our dialogue with the nineras, at last feeling like we were connecting, Friar Guillermo came gliding into our little corner, long brown robes flowing behind him, hands clasped together at the waist. Behind him was a camera crew from the Channel 7 Eye-Witness News in Guatemala City. Spanish flew everywhere as the nineras jumped up and started bustling around. We were swirled into the treatment room, children placed on equipment and with toys, lights were lit and they started filming. Perplexed, I did the best I could to offer children I had never met, and with whom I could not speak, some kind of appropriate handling. It is said that Guatemalan officials do not like to acknowledge the existence of so much starvation in their country, so this could be seen as a political statement on the part of the news and the Friar. So ended the first class.

As I worked with the women of the nutritional recovery program, I learned about starvation. As the body starves, it shuts down all unnecessary activities, including response to outside stimulation. The Merck Manual (1987) calls it petulant apathy, referring to both the lack of interest in life and the irritability of the children. We know through research how important the first few years are for getting stimulation into growing little minds (White, 1975). Judith and the nineras showed me that movement and touch, primary means of stimulating babies, became almost intolerable to a starving infant. As they begin to recover, a pincer grasp and hand to mouth movement may be the first movement pattern to appear in a child over twelve months. This surprised me, as I had always assumed that the neurodevelopmental principle of proximal control being necessary to distal accuracy (Boehme, 1988) was universal to movement problems. Perhaps because these patterns had already developed, they were available to the older infant and called upon first due to their survival value. Certainly the children who could use only these patterns relied on the surface support to move by sliding their arms along the mat. Exploration of the environment and play with gross motor patterns, which we in the United States consider critical to early child development are a long time in coming. So is language development (Photo 3).

To my delight, the traditional culture of Guatemala has an excellent solution to stimulating movement and touch in the wearing of the rebozos or large shawls to carry around young children. I was pleased to wear one around and discover that by moving playfully myself, I was able to give the young ones a great deal of quality stimulation. Mayan women are already using the shawls and I encouraged the Ladino nineras to adopt them in the center. Realistically, they probably won't wear them, but the acknowledgement of the value of the reboza may lend dignity to the Mayan women working there.

Language stimulation was a little trickier because the nineras knew no Spanish nursery rhymes and their children's songs were long and complex. Judith translated "Head, shoulders, knees and toes" into Spanish and we started a morning circle time with the children.

Judith had concerns about using the Peabody Developmental Motor Scales (Folio and Fewell, 1983) with the children as I had urged her to do. She felt it was too culturally biased. I resisted the idea, thinking that motor skills are motor skills, and not subject to the same problems that a language or cognitive scale might be. We gave the Peabody to some of the children in the Nutritional Recovery program. It changed my mind. Children who have never had the exposure to peg boards, form boards, scissors or blocks, can not be accurately assessed for their motor capabilities with typical North

PHOTO 3. Nutritional Recovery Staff member uses a shawl to hold a sensitive infant.

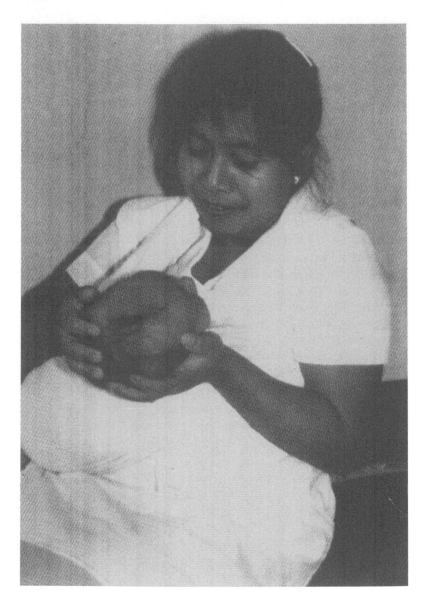

American developmental assessments. Because these children are just gaining imitation skills and mechanical manipulation of tools is a rarer experience for them, the Peabody becomes an assessment of the early cognitive function of learning through imitation instead of an assessment of motor functioning. It is far more accurate to observe spontaneous play, looking for motor patterns such as the ability to release in space using a pincer grasp, and tool use with a spoon, observing for finger tip prehension and supination, than to use standardized tests.

My reading before going to Guatemala had included a book by Bruno Bettleheim called "The Good Enough Parent" (1987). His insight about the nature of instruction proved valuable to me. He pointed out that how-to instructions are somewhat helpful when assembling inanimate objects, like a home barbecue, but they are a hindrance when dealing with people. With a barbecue, one has a general idea of just how the object should turn out. And when following the directions, if one gets lost or frustrated, one can always put them aside and start again later. However, when dealing with people, no two situations are ever the same. Simple formulas and step-by-step instructions are rarely applicable, and when they do have relevance, often the consumer of such information either cannot remember all the steps or applies them in a stilted manner. Bettleheim calls for adults working with children to do so from an empathetic point of view, developing a vision of qualities to be enhanced in each child according to that child's unique assets.

As therapists we face a similar task to that of parenting. We want to look at each child's unique blend of personality and interests when working to develop their skills. It is also critical for us to understand the fundamental underlying principles that allow for function. In the case of the children at the Casa, it was clear that movement patterns, reactivity to sensory stimulation, and development of problem solving skills were all principles that staff needed to understand. I was concerned that if I taught by giving step-by-step formulas, the staff would never be able to apply the teachings once I was gone. What I wanted to impart was the underlying principles that needed to be worked on. This was especially important to me when working with the therapists (Photo 4).

Our routine in the therapy department was to meet at noon for a

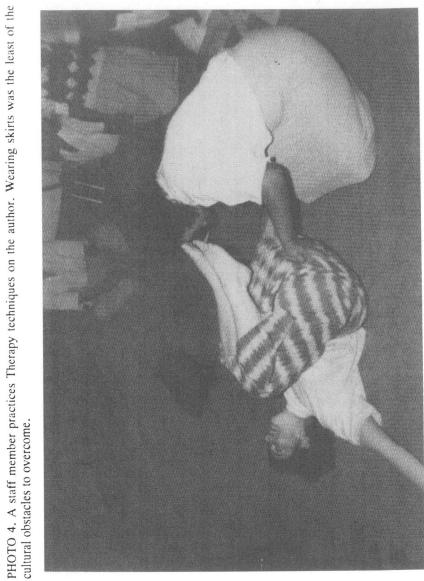

PHOTO 4. A staff member practices Therapy techniques on the author. Wearing skirts was the least of the cultural obstacles to overcome.

ninety-minute class. They designed the course so that each day was a case presentation during which I would talk through what I was observing and then attempt a treatment session. The rest of the time I would then have them practice the therapy techniques, expanding their skills as we practiced on each other.

Oscar, the physical therapist trained in Costa Rica, was fun to watch. He had read of many of the techniques of the Bobaths and heard of them in his lectures, but had never seen them demonstrated. Though he spoke no English, the words I used were familiar to him and his eyes would often light up even before Judith translated. His staff was mostly young high school graduates. Since most children drop out of school after third grade to work, these young people represented the small educated middle class of the country. To work for Oscar, they had to do extensive reading and study hard. I found them to be earnest and skillful in their work (Photo 5).

One day mid-week of the first week, the therapists presented a sixteen-year-old boy with spastic quadriplegic cerebral palsy. David was able to sit up in a wheelchair and all agreed that he seemed to be quite intelligent and motivated. If only they could break up some of the spasticity in his hands so he could participate in the school programs or the sheltered workshop activities. Handling him, I found that given stability, his tone reduced nicely. Looking at his severely pronated feet and his internally rotated, fisted hands, I knew where he had been gaining his stability all of his life. He had tightened the only parts he could control to keep his body somehow stabilized in an upright position. I treated him, gently inhibiting extensor tone and stretching what I could. As he gained midline trunk control, his hands opened up, and then we put him in his wheelchair.

Sitting in the adult sized wheelchair, this small young man's hips went into hyperextension on the loose sling seat and back. To compensate and stay upright, he did the only thing he could do, he curved his upper back forward and then hyperextended his neck to look forward. A familiar pattern to those of us treating cerebral palsy, but it undid all the work I had just done.

I asked the therapists if the carpenter could make a firm seat and back insert. The carpenters are on the premises to repair the build-

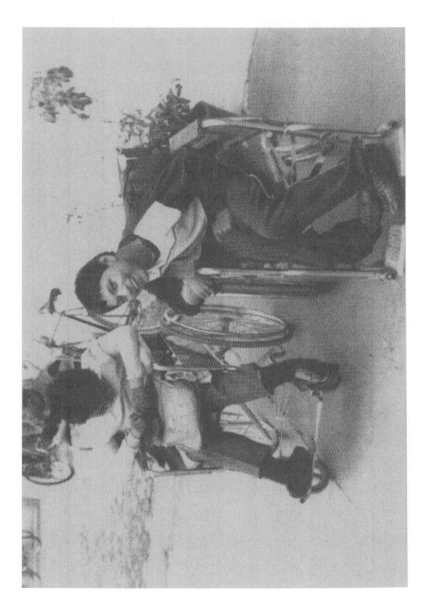

PHOTO 5. David in his wheelchair.

ing, not to make equipment for the children, they said. Certainly there must be something we could do, I maintained. No one among the staff thought so. However, a retired lady from Florida who had sat in on the class that day thought she could smuggle in used wheelchairs from Florida, there certainly being a surplus of wheelchairs in that state. Duty, she reasoned, would have to be paid on each chair if she just sent them directly. But if everyone we knew could enter Guatemala with a bandaged leg, requiring a wheelchair to move around, no duty could be charged. Annoyed as I was by the rescuer from the North mentality, (I wanted the solutions to come locally to ensure they would be continued) it still tickled my funny bone to contemplate the stream of gringos coming in from Miami in wheelchairs (Photo 6).

Walking out of the Casa for lunch that day, I walked through a ward of severely involved children, laid out in the sun on mats. Their bodies twisted from years of extensor muscles going unopposed in their pull. Then I walked past the office where the secretary was proudly using her new computer. The Fax machine sat next to her. Lots of foreigners passed through Antigua, and those who found their way to the Casa were often moved to want to help. Their gifts reflected their knowledge of what could be useful. Hence the modern office, the new van, even the tons of stuffed animals Judith was always receiving. But did anyone know how powerful the funds to hire a local carpenter for the therapists could be? The therapists themselves had no idea of what could be accomplished with some simple positioning devices.

It felt like only I had any idea of how much improved the situation could be by training local people to help themselves. David could develop hand function if he was properly stabilized. His life could be far more rewarding. I envisioned what he would have been like if he had grown up in the United States and I wanted to create a better system at the Casa. And the more severely involved kids, even if we could only get them sitting up in proper chairs, could look around instead of always at the ceiling. Their extensor tone reduced, leg adductors would not be so tight, they would be easier to feed, change and care for, making carrying and transferring easier. No one knew this at the Casa. How could they know what to ask for when they did not know the possibilities?

PHOTO 6. The children with severe involvement from years of poor positioning.

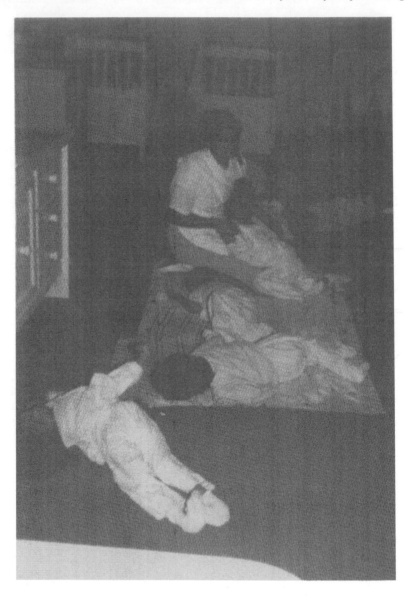

After lunch, I went and spoke to the medical director. Judith warned me that he would find no solution. It was true. Somehow, it was not possible to pay a carpenter, or pay for wood, and what about tools. I asked if there was room at the Casa for a woodworking shop. Yes. I thought for a bit. Certainly I could get tools donated back in the United States. But what about paying the carpenter and buying wood? Well, I can not imagine it would be all that expensive in American dollars to fund such a program; I am sure I could work it out. (Careful, Judith warned me, you are already overstretched at home, do not offer more than you think you can really do.) (But how could I let the children down?)

In retrospect, I realize that it was to the doctor's advantage to downplay any possible homegrown solutions and wait to see just what I might be able to offer. Many of the activities and environments that Judith has created at the Casa have been imitated and developed further when staff members there have had a chance to see a model at work. She is almost never acknowledged directly as the source of inspiration, yet place after place in the Casa has been transformed to be quite like what she has initiated. Though the Casa never has many funds, they have found ways to make things happen, from the ten new teachers to the stars and moons hanging from the ceiling in the children's bedrooms. If I had had the time, simple modeling of constructing adaptive equipment might have been the best solution. Unfortunately, I had two weeks and felt a sense of urgency.

Soon I was telling Oscar about my plans. I began talking with people knowledgeable in woodworking. They warned me that wood was very expensive in Guatemala, and the quality of it was poor. Guatemalan carpenters, they told me, were generally unskilled. None of this bothered me. I felt full of the rightness of my mission, and certain that things would work out because it was so right.

Over the weekend, Judith and I took a trip to a lovely Inn on the banks of Lake Atitlan. On Sunday I was sitting on the veranda eating breakfast when Judith found me, writing a list of things I needed to do for my carpenter project. Quietly, with great deliberation and seriousness, she sat down and said she must speak to me. I had never experienced foreboding and dread in the presence of my dear friend before, but I sure did then. Judith started talking about the misgivings she was having about the carpenter project. Sara, she said, who is going to administer this project? Well, Oscar of course. I would train him to understand positioning better and he would design the equipment and direct the carpenter. He would have the "Disabled Village Children" in Spanish as a constant guide. But Sara, this is your vision. We do not know what Oscar wants for himself, how long he plans to work for the Casa. He could make a lot more money as a private therapist in Guatemala City.

The conflict in me was incredibly painful. The rightness of the project meshed with a part of me that still wanted to rescue these people. My developing value of working with therapy consumers in a way that allowed their values and goals to lead seemingly contradicted my pursuing the carpenter project. In North America, without the language and cultural barriers, I still could have come in conflict with these two opposing forces. As professionals, we are taught that we hold the vision, the clinical understanding, the expertise to know what should happen. As helping professionals, we have a strong drive to make better any suffering we see. And yet, as occupational therapists, we know that the will and drive, the intrinsic motivation to act, must come from within the client or system we are assisting. Our goal is always to facilitate the development of their strengths and visions, not to impose our own.

Judith painfully broke the ice. She asked me if I was angry with her. I was furious with her for bringing this up, yet I loved her integrity and she was right. In my panic I could see no middle ground. We started to talk it out and eventually agreed to back off a bit. It might mean my reapproaching the medical director and having to explain my overenthusiastic beginnings but we needed to be sure the vision was theirs. So we decided to invite Oscar to tea.

Oscar came to tea Monday evening. As the conversation unfolded, he told us how he had come to be a physical therapist. He had originally volunteered at the Casa while in high school, thinking to some day be a physical education teacher. Working with the missionary/therapist, the plight of the children there moved him greatly. Friar Guillermo had come to understand the need for a physical therapist. He sent Oscar to Costa Rica to study, paying his tuition and having him stay with the Friar's mother. In exchange,

Oscar was working for free until the Friar could find the funds to pay him. Oscar then told us of his hopes to go to the therapy school run by Americans in Cuernovaca, Mexico, where Christine Nelson OTR is an NDT instructor. He had heard they had a program there for Latin American therapists that would train him in better handling techniques. It was his intention to continue indefinitely at the Casa. So Oscar was living at home, working for free, supervising a therapy department at the age of twenty-three. Most men his age would still be living at home, but they would be contributing financially.

I told Oscar that I had been hasty in jumping in, wanting to create an equipment shop. I saw now that my first priority should be to help him if I could in getting to the NDT course in Cuernovaca. There, I told him, he would learn about positioning and equipment and develop his own vision. He would gain a far clearer picture of what materials and construction methods would be appropriate in his area than I could possibly ever have. I told him I would very much like to continue our friendship and assist him in developing his vision by getting tools, or doing consultation and trainings or any other way he could think of.

I went back to the medical director and told him that before we could start an equipment shop, Oscar needed further training so that he would know how to best use its resources. I assured him that if the Casa could help Oscar to get to Cuernovaca, that they would have made a very wise investment indeed.

Perhaps other therapists would have responded to this situation with more moderation and political savvy. But my observations of Americans in Guatemala was that we all tended to be drawn into trying to "save" people there. And we all had expectations of getting in and acting quickly, wanting to immediately jump into problem solving. Even people who were not novices in the culture like me, got swept away with grand schemes. The retired lady who wanted to smuggle in wheelchairs rather than looking for a sustainable local solution, had been working in Latin America for years.

The clash between my own ethics and my style of doing things was a turning point for me. I look at the way I work with parents and systems back in the United States with more of an eye for avoiding the drama of fixing things for people. I value to a greater degree the notion of helping people to define for themselves what it is that they want. Often I have a vision of possibilities they do not yet perceive. I know how to proceed, the methods to use, that they do not know about. But even with (or perhaps especially with) a two-year-old, I watch actions and listen to ideas, deciphering what it is that the child is wanting to accomplish and experience. I am constantly holding two visions for my clients and families. One vision is to assist people in organizing their actions to attain their goals. The other vision is of the long-term potentials that because of my experience I may have a clearer picture of.

It sounds so simple. It is the essence of occupational therapy; the activities one chooses, or the manner in which one sets up the activity are designed to produce more healing as they accomplish the short-term goals of the client. Be it introducing a bilateral component to the play of a two-year-old with hemiplegia, or the idea that positioning will sustain gains made in therapy, introducing potentials and letting the client choose them as their own is a sustainable way to interact therapeutically.

The rest of the visit was far more peaceful for me. Staff in the Casa continued to be shy and found it awkward to touch each other during practice sessions. Over time I found ways to joke and clown, even with very poor Spanish. In the end, I too have become a story teller and adventurer. I even smuggled a nun's tumour back into the States. But that is another story.

REFERENCES

Acker, A. (1986). *Children of the Volcano.* Westport, CT: Lawrence Hill & Co.

Bettelheim, B. (1987). *A good enough parent.* New York: Random House.

Boehme, R. (1988). *Improving upper body control.* Tucson: Therapy Skill Builders.

Folio, M. & Fewell, R. (1983). *Peabody developmental motor scales.* Allen, Texas: DLM Teaching Resources.

Growing Old Fast in Guatemala. (1991, January). *New York Times Magazine* p. 20-23.

Guatemala: Axel Mejia, Street Educator. (1990, December). Urgent Action Bulletin.

The Merck Manual, 13th Ed. (1987). Kwashiorkor. Rahway: Merck and Co. pp. 1149-1151.

Oetter, P. (1984). Sensory Integration: Treatment applications, workshop manual. Torrance, CA: Sensory Integration International.

Werner, D. (1985). *Helping health workers learn*. Palo Alto, CA: Hesperian Foundation.

Werner, D. (1987). *Disabled village children*. Palo Alto, CA: Hesperian Foundation.

White, B. (1975). *The first three years of life*. Englewood Cliffs, NJ: Prentice-Hall, Inc.

Sensory Integration in Finland

Betsy A. Slavik, MA, OTR

SUMMARY. This article describes the development and organization of a sensory integration training course given in Finland. Facts that impact on the success of international health education are discussed in relation to the model used for this course. In addition, cultural differences (e.g., language, customs, health care, and education systems) are discussed as they relate to this teaching experience and to occupational therapy practice in Finland. The summary highlights examples of how teaching and/or working in another culture can impact on professional development.

INTRODUCTION

In the summer of 1985, a long awaited 3-month sensory integration course was given in Finland. The seed for this course was planted years ago in 1980, while both Paivi Danner, M.A., O.T. (a Finnish occupational therapist) and I were graduate students at the University of Southern California, and completing a four-month post-graduate course with A. Jean Ayres, Ph.D., O.T.R. This article will describe the development and organization of the sensory integration course, as well as give insight into the practice of occupational therapy in Finland.

First, it is important to understand the background of Finland and

Betsy A. Slavik is the Occupational Therapy Consultant for the San Diego and Imperial Counties Developmental Services, Inc. Her address is: San Diego Regional Center, 4355 Ruffin Road, Suite 206, San Diego, CA 92123.

This manuscript is dedicated in memory to A.J. Ayres, PhD, OTR, for her life's work which has greatly influenced the evolution of occupational therapy practice. Special thanks goes to Paivi Danner, MA, OT, a friend and colleague whose hard work and dedication made this course possible. Lastly, I would like to mention the Finnish occupational therapists who demonstrated a strong desire to learn, and yet were able to balance work, play, and leisure.

39

its people, and the history of occupational therapy education and practice. Finland is an independent country of Northern Europe and is typically referred to as a Scandinavian country. Like the United States, Finland has a fairly high standard of living. Its economy has traditionally centered on vast timber resources, however, since 1944 new industries such as shipbuilding and metal working have developed. Also since World War II and the rapid post-war industrialization, there has been a population shift from rural to urban areas (Random House, 1983).

The Finnish government is a Democratic Republic and the people elect the President and Parliament. The chief cities are in the southern, more coastal areas of the country, with Helsinki, the capital, being the largest with a population of approximately 497,000. More than 90% of the population speaks Finnish and about 7% speak Swedish. Both languages are official languages in Finland (Random House, 1983). English and German are common third languages taught in Finnish schools.

Finland, and other Scandinavian countries, are known for their progressive attitudes about the importance of health and social welfare programs that promote the health and development of families. The people of these countries continue to vote in high tax rates to fund these programs (40-50% of gross income for middle class families). When compared with the United States, these countries have significantly lower rates for births of low-weight babies, perinatal and infant mortality, induced abortion, adolescent pregnancy, and child abuse (Chamberlin, 1990).

Occupational therapy is a recently established group in Finland. The first class of occupational therapists graduated in the early 1970's. The educational program was organized from a European model; that is, occupational therapy is a 3-year college program. Finland has not yet established occupational therapy as a 4-year university degree program. The colleges do offer 1-year courses in specialty areas, e.g., pediatrics. According to Ms. Danner (1991), occupational therapists in Finland have been working toward establishing a graduate degree program through the university system. The opportunity will be available for occupational therapists to obtain what is equivalent to the United States' Master's and Doctoral degrees.

A population that Finnish occupational therapists commonly work with is children with minimal brain dysfunction (MBD). Minimal brain dysfunction is a term that has been used to describe a group of children who are non-retarded, non-cerebral palsied, and showing signs of minor neurological dysfunctions and attentional deficits (Kohler & Regeflak, 1973-78). The term "learning disabilities" is not used before a child enters school, which in Finland is at the age of 7. Historically, the treatment of children with MBD in Finland was influenced by neuro-developmental therapy, perceptual motor approaches, and play therapy (Danner, 1983). According to Ms. Danner (1983), a question arose as to the effectiveness of these approaches alone to address the neurological problems identified in children with MBD. Sensory integration was thought to offer promise as it had in the United States and Australia. With this in mind, Ms. Danner came to the University of Southern California to obtain her Master's degree and to study sensory integration. That is how I met her and became involved in the project for the study of sensory integration in Finland.

Sensory integration refers to the process of organizing sensory information in the brain for the purpose of accomplishing self-directed, meaningful activity (Ayres, 1979). Over a course of more than 20 years, Dr. A.J. Ayres developed the theory of sensory integration, which refers to the concepts and principles related to central nervous system functioning and development. When applying theory to practice, Dr. Ayres also developed what is referred to as sensory integrative procedures for treatment, as well as a standardized tool for the identification of sensory integrative dysfunction. The Southern California Sensory Integration Test (SCSIT) was the original battery of tests, which have since been expanded and re-standardized as the Sensory Integration and Praxis Tests (SIPT). In the United States, there is a certification procedure for the administration and interpretation of the tests, but no standardized training procedure for treatment.

At the time of the course in Finland, both Paivi Danner and I had completed the four-month, post-graduate course with Dr. A.J. Ayres and were certified in the administration and interpretation of the SCSIT. In addition, I had worked approximately 3 years as a part-time staff therapist at the Ayres Clinic and was involved in the re-standardization project of the SIPT.

COURSE ORGANIZATION

According to health education experts (Williams, Baumslag, & Jelliffe, 1985), health education is most likely to be successful if it is planned in the local cultural framework. They further state that attitudes of health professionals can effect the success of the educational process. Professionals should speak the same language, empathize and respect those they are trying to educate.

In laying the foundation for support of sensory integrative theory and treatment in Finland, Paivi Danner, along with guidance from Dr. A. Jean Ayres and others, decided an effective approach would be to: (1) return home and do an effectiveness study on Finnish children as her Master's thesis; (2) slowly begin to introduce the theory and treatment principles via lectures to physicians, therapists, educators, and parents; and (3) translate the book *Sensory Integration and The Child* by A.J. Ayres into Finnish. This approach proved to be effective in gaining professional support to eventually obtain financial support to sponsor a 3-month course.

In 1981, I took a brief vacation to Finland which gave me an introduction to its geography, people, and customs. During 1982-83, Paivi Danner and I wrote a grant proposal to the Finnish National Board of Vocational Education and the Finnish College of Health Sciences to obtain financial support for a 3-month sensory integration training course for Finnish occupational therapists. Initially the cost of the course was felt to be too high by the funding agencies. However, with continued support, especially from the Health Administration Department, the National Board of Vocational Education and the Finnish College of Health Sciences approved the course with some changes in the original plan. The primary change was from our initial plan to limit enrollment to six, to the final allowance of 12-15. Our initial plan was to have a significant amount of clinical experience, which with 12-15 therapists would be more limited. However, we both felt that the primary goals of the course could still be met. This leads to how we viewed the purpose of a 3-month course.

The primary purpose was to give the Finnish occupational therapists an introduction to sensory integration theory, testing procedures, and treatment. We hoped to give a better understanding of the theory and its use; to build a foundation for learning; and to stimulate interest in continuing to expand that foundation of knowledge.

The lecture portion of the course took place at Kuopio University in Kuopio, Finland. The clinical component took place at both the University Hospital Children's Clinic in Kuopio and Lastenlinna Children's Hospital in Helsinki. The three-month course met 5 days per week, between 8-10 hours each day. Twelve occupational therapists were selected. Priority was given to those who had completed the one-year specialty in pediatrics. In addition, because I do not speak Finnish, another qualification was the ability to read and speak English. All 12 therapists had at some time heard Paivi Danner lecture on sensory integration theory and all were instructed to have read *Sensory Integration and The Child* and to have reviewed basic neurophysiology of the sensory systems prior to the course. It should be noted that most employers fully financed participation in the course.

We approached organizing and teaching the course in what we felt was a logical, developmental sequence for learning. A decision was made to have some of the technical lectures given in Finnish. We utilized neurologists, audiologists, and psychologists from the community to teach portions of the neuro-science lectures and statistics. This also served to facilitate interest and support of the course from the local health professional community. The basic components of the course included:

1. Neuro-science lectures including the relationship to sensory systems dysfunction;
2. Beginning theory, including historical perspective;
3. Test and measurements including statistics, test development, test mechanics, clinical observation, interpretation, and report writing. (Test mechanics were observed prior to testing normal children and again during testing of dysfunctional children; interpretation was done throughout the last two months.);
4. Normal sensory-motor development, cognitive development and play;
5. Advanced theory;

6. Advanced study of specific types of sensory integrative dysfunctions;
7. Art of therapy, adaptive response, sensory integrative therapy principles and treatment activities;
8. How to measure effectiveness of treatment; and
9. Clinical experience which included further observation of testing, additional interpretation, and actual one-to-one clinical experience with treatment.

TEACHING EXPERIENCE

Because of the language difference, I had planned to supplement my lectures with audio-visual aids. I came equipped with numerous slides and videos. Because the European video system is different than the United States', all videos had to be transferred. After the first day, I quickly realized that my outlines for lectures had to be very specific and therefore, lengthy. This meant many long evening hours of preparation for me, but allowed the therapists more freedom to listen and watch without having to worry about writing extensive notes. Language did occasionally pose a difficulty during lectures, but fortunately Paivi Danner was usually available for translation. It is interesting to note here that many of our therapy "jargon" terms were not able to be translated directly into Finnish. Also, there were occasions when a word or words were used to define a concept in which there were not similar words for the therapists to attach meaning in their language. For example, when discussing the timing and sequencing of movements in relation to motor planning and praxis, there were no similar terms in Finnish for "timing" and "sequencing." Therefore, the terms had to be described and when "timing" and "sequencing" were then used in lectures, therapists had a concept to attach to these words.

Occasionally, there were misconceptions about American culture and lifestyle. I remember one time when discussing treatment planning, a therapist spoke up and commented that scheduling sometimes poses difficulty because, unlike in America, many Finnish women have to work. With further discussion, it was interesting to find out that many of their concepts of American life come from television ("Dallas" was a popular show on Finnish television), and from newspapers, magazines and books. Many of the therapists were also under the impression that the United States had no health and financial aid plans for the poor. In a country with strong national health and social welfare programs, our system can seem insufficient. I mention this only because these situations made me further appreciate the effects of media on our understanding and conceptions of other cultures.

In addition to use of a wide variety of visual and audio/visual aids in teaching, health education experts recommended the use of teaching aids developed within and/or by the local community (Williams et al. 1985). Numerous videotapes were made throughout the course of treatment demonstrations, use of clinical observations in assessment, and of every child's initial therapy session. These videos proved valuable for later discussion and treatment planning, and were left with the Finnish therapists for future study. In addition, many of the children were to continue in treatment so the tapes could be used as a data base for measuring effectiveness of therapy.

CLINICAL EXPERIENCE

During the clinical treatment sessions, language did not pose a barrier. Families were very receptive to having an "American guest therapist" work with their child. The children were wonderful. I was somewhat of a novelty. It was enlightening to see how efficient gestures, facial expressions, and one-to-two word utterances were as means of communication. When I returned home, I was much more aware of the amount, type, and speed of communication I use during therapy sessions.

Children were referred for testing primarily by pediatricians and pediatric neurologists. If the test results indicated a sensory integrative dysfunction, the child was placed in the clinical/treatment portion of the course. Paivi Danner had translated the directions of the Southern California Sensory Integration Test (1978) for the therapists, and trained them in its development, administration, and interpretation. The decision was made to use the SCSIT for several reasons. First, reportedly preliminary pilot studies of other American standardized tests indicated Finnish children perform similarly. Secondly, the Finnish therapists plan to begin their own pilot studies of normative data comparison. Lastly, no other tests were available to the Finnish therapists to begin identifying sensory integrative dysfunction.

Most of the children in the course came from the local city area and up to a one-hour drive away. My understanding is that children are frequently referred to the Pediatric Rehabilitation Department of the Children's Hospital/Clinic for in-depth work-ups to identify and clarify the nature of their developmental delays, learning, and/or behavior problems. The team assessment can include neurology, psychology, speech, occupational therapy, and physical therapy. Because of the rural nature of Finland, children are admitted for up to 3 weeks for completion of these diagnostics and implementation of a program plan. Several of the children in our course were in-patients at the Children's Hospital. Most of the children were between 5 and 8 years of age, although there were a few between 3-5 years of age.

As mentioned previously, two clinical sites were utilized, one in Kuopio and the other in Helsinki. A group of twelve students were divided into three groups of four. Two groups completed the two-week clinical portion in Kuopio, and one in Helsinki. The two-week clinical consisted of 3 hours of individual treatment 5 days per week, afternoon case reviews and discussions, with 1-2 evaluations per week. I supervised the group in Helsinki as well as co-supervised one group in Kuopio. Because Paivi Danner had been providing occupational therapy utilizing a sensory integrative approach at her clinic in Kuopio, that clinic was well-equipped for the clinical practice. The occupational therapy department at the Children's Hospital in Helsinki designed a clinic specifically for the course. Equipment is even more expensive to obtain in Finland because of the customs/import charges, which can often raise the cost by 20-30%. Therefore, most of the suspended equipment, climbing structures, barrels, ramp, scooter boards, trapezes, and large pillows were made by the engineering department at the hospital. Some pieces of equipment were also made by an occupational therapist who has started a small therapy equipment business in Finland. The equipment was all well made, and the suspension systems were designed to hold a 1,500 pound workload.

LIVING ENVIRONMENT

As mentioned previously, Finland and the United States have a high standard of living in common. What was particularly striking was that poverty appeared virtually non-existent both in urban and rural areas. Government subsidized housing was clean and well maintained.

During my stay in Kuopio, I lived in a rental apartment approximately half a mile from Kuopio University and several miles from the Children's Clinic. I usually walked to and from the course, although public transportation was excellent. In Helsinki, I rented a room in an apartment of a therapist in the course, which was approximately a 30 minute ride to the Children's Hospital. I learned to take a variety of methods of transportation, i.e., train, trolley, bus. Because the Finnish language does not have a common Latin base, I had to rely on landmarks to orient me geographically and pictures on packages and bottles to identify foods. A typical street sign could be 20 letters long.

In general, my impression was that the Finnish people live simply and do not waste. Most items such as food and clothing are very expensive, therefore people have to be careful about what they buy. The overall environment was very clean and poverty as we see here in the United States was virtually nonexistent. Europeans tend to have a different routine than Americans, both in mealtime and work schedules. Most workdays begin at 8:30 or 9:00 a.m. Midmorning breaks are common, and the afternoon meal is the primary hot meal of the day. During the summer months, the daylight hours are long (18-20 hours), so either you become accustomed to sleeping while it's light or adjust to fewer hours of sleep. I must say that I found my living conditions to be comfortable and the Finnish people, as a group, friendly. I thoroughly enjoyed experiencing some of the customs, e.g., the early morning open air markets and saunas.

COURSE EFFECTIVENESS

To assist with ongoing course development and future planning, we did attempt to evaluate course effectiveness through question/

answer periods throughout the course, a structured non-graded post test, and a course evaluation questionnaire. From all of these methods, we were able to identify strengths and weaknesses of the course, as well as areas for continuing education. The therapists acknowledged an increased awareness of the importance of research and the need for continual study to expand their knowledge of this therapeutic program. Additional feedback since the course completion has been the continued support and encouragement the therapists receive from physicians, parents, and other professionals. Many of the therapists who initially did not have adequate treatment facilities for sensory integration procedures have since been given the space and equipment.

OCCUPATIONAL THERAPY PRACTICE

In touring the Children's Hospital in Helsinki, which is the country's largest, it was interesting to note that the occupational therapists each had their own office on their particular unit, e.g., rehabilitation in-patient, out-patient, acute. Treatment was carried out in the offices which tended to be about 10' by 12'-14' in size. In general, each office contained a desk, bookshelf, testing table, and fine motor play area. This arrangement typified the traditional orientation of occupational therapy in Finland. There was no large general joint treatment area. There was one small joint therapy room, however, it could not accommodate large movement activities. The clinic space designed for the sensory integration course was borrowed from physical therapy.

In regards to occupational therapy practice in Finland, it was also noted that productivity was at around 3-4 hrs. per day. Because of the national health care system, occupational therapy is reportedly available to all who require it. Occupational therapy did not appear to have the strict documentation, productivity, and quality assurance guidelines that are required in the United States. Chamberlin (1990) discussed the differences in health care in Scandinavian countries from the United States. He stated that the Scandinavian countries do not talk about cost effectiveness of programs. The services are provided because they are seen as important support systems for families and children. This trend might be changing as seen by individuals and families supplementing health care with private plans. Upon subsequent visits to Finland, I noted an increased number of occupational therapists in private practice.

My previous clinical experience prior to the course included two years of practice in a Neonatal Intensive Care Unit (NICU). As part of the course, I presented a lecture and clinical field experience on the topic of occupational therapy practice in the NICU. The chief neonatologist at the University Hospital in Kuopio was very supportive of occupational therapy intervention. At the time, occupational therapy practice was primarily aimed at children 3 years and above. Occupational therapy was not involved in infant care. However, the occupational therapists in the course were very interested in learning more about the areas of NICU and early intervention services.

Because of the evolutionary status of occupational therapy in Finland, it appears that they rely on other countries for initial knowledge and training in specialty areas, e.g., neuro-developmental therapy, sensory integration, early intervention. Like in the United States, occupational therapy in Finland also struggles with recognition and lack of understanding of the field. It appears that occupational therapy education not being a part of the university system, has an impact on its status as a health care field. During my stay, I was asked to speak at a national conference of pediatric neurologists, to a group of neuro-psychologists, and to the pediatric staff at Children's Hospital, Helsinki. The purpose of these presentations was to support sensory integration education and practice in Finland and promote the understanding of occupational therapy. The issues that seem to influence the development of professional status can include the responsibility of managing self, achieving a level of autonomy and the level of terminal university degree. It is clear that as occupational therapy evolves in Finland, these issues are being addressed.

In continuing education supported by the Finnish government, Finnish Occupational Therapy Association, and employers of occupational therapists, the long-term goal is to have Finnish therapists trained to enable them to teach courses locally. Following the 1985 sensory integration course, the original twelve occupational therapists and Paivi Danner began meeting one day per month to review and clarify all course information, to discuss specific case studies, and to explore methods for effective and appropriate documentation of assessment and treatment. Since the initial course, the Finnish therapists have planned and completed two additional three-month courses, which have resulted in approximately 36 occupational therapists with advanced training in sensory integration.

I was invited back to Finland to lecture on two separate occasions. The first invitation was in 1986 by the Children's Hospital of Helsinki for a week-long series of lectures on early intervention. In 1989, I was again invited to return and present a two-week advanced sensory integration treatment course for all occupational therapists who had completed the 3-month course. On each occasion, I experienced mutual respect, friendliness, and a shared willingness to question and learn.

CONCLUSION

This article illustrates a model for the transference of knowledge from one culture to another. Although there are many similarities between Finland and the United States, differences exist that do influence the acceptance and assimilation of information. Some of the differences highlighted in this article include language, customs, health care and reimbursement systems, and educational systems.

Responses of therapists during and immediately following the course, as well as from subsequent continuing education plans, indicate that the initial sensory integration training course was a success. The single most important factor in the success would seem to be that it occurred within the local cultural framework. In other words, Paivi Danner, being from the country and knowledgeable in sensory integration theory, assessment and treatment was therefore able to facilitate great interest and lay a strong foundation of support. Other factors contributing to the success included: a shared investment of the instructors in sensory integration education and training; sufficient length of course which allowed for creative adaptations of teaching methods and insuring thoroughness; involvement of professionals from local health care and educational community in technical aspects of training; sufficient financial support for therapists to attend a comprehensive, in-depth training; and the openness in communication and mutual respect between instructors and therapists.

I doubt if anyone can come away from an experience of living, teaching, and/or working in another country without it having a profound impact on both their personal and professional lives. My present job involves working with a variety of ethnic groups of various socio-economic status. I am much more aware of speaking slowly; using simple, non-jargon terminology in my explanations, and more sensitive to the impact of non-verbal communication during assessment, therapy, and conferences.

Attempting to gain a better understanding of another country's health, education, and social welfare systems has given me a greater realization of the complexity of our systems and the amount of information families must integrate. Not only do we have federal programs, but also state and local programs that many families need to access. With our transient society, a family can encounter differences between, as well as within a state. I am now more sensitive to my responsibility in assisting families to make informed choices.

The teaching experience encouraged me, and in some cases necessitated, that I explore creative, alternative methods of instruction. The use of clinical demonstrations and videos developed with the local community were extremely effective.

Lastly, I came away from this experience with an increased appreciation of the evolution of occupational therapy in the United States, and a feeling of pride about our professional commitment to grow, expand, and strengthen our foundation. I see it happen daily in the clinic, as well as through our educational programs and research efforts. The commitment is evident in the United States at the grassroots, state, and national levels of our professional organizations. My experience with the Finnish occupational therapists further substantiated how committed individuals working together can make a difference.

BIBLIOGRAPHY

Ayres, A.J. (1979). *Sensory integration and the child*. Los Angeles: Western Psychological Services.

Chamberlin, R. (1990). *Community wide approaches to promoting the health and development of families with children: Examples from Scandinavia and Great Britain*. Public Health 655, Section 2, San Diego State University.

Danner, P. (1983). *Effectiveness of sensory integrative procedures on four Finnish preschoolers with minimal brain dysfunction*. Unpublished master's thesis, University of Southern California, Los Angeles.

Danner, P. (1991). *Personal communication*. March.

Kohler, E.M., & Regeflak, C. (1973-78). *Minimal Brain Dysfunction in Preschool-At Risk for Trouble in School?* Pediatrician, 219-227.

Mitchell, J. (1983). *Random house encyclopedia*. N Y: Random House.

Williams, C.D., Baumslag, N., & Jelliffe, D.B. (1985). *Mother and child health, delivering the services*. London: Oxford University Press.

Schizophrenia:
Living with Madness
Here and in Zanzibar

Juli Evans, MSEd, BS, OTR

SUMMARY. In Zanzibar, as in many "third world" places, there are two health care systems, one traditional and the other "European." Among the Swahili people of East Africa spirits are believed to be the cause of disturbed behavior or "madness." Data and observations gathered during one year of mental health practice in Zanzibar and over many years of practice in the U.S. are compared to examine how cultural values shape beliefs, practices and attitudes related to "madness." Implications for occupational therapy theory and practice are drawn.

INTRODUCTION

Sometimes it becomes necessary to curse them, when you have reached that final stage, then you tell them that you do not want to be bothered with them, then sometimes you decide to curse them. Then maybe they will be quiet.

R.A., 25 years old, female, citizen of Zanzibar, Tanzania

Juli Evans is a Professor in the School of Occupational Therapy and Physical Therapy at the University of Puget Sound, 1500 North Warner Street, Tacoma, WA 98416.

The author wishes to thank the staff of the Kidongo Chekundu Mental Hospital and of the Ministry of Health, particularly Dr. Abdulwakil Idrissa Abdulwakil, Mr. Ahmed Awadh Salim, Dr. Sixten Bondestam, and Dr. Joop Garssen. In addition she is grateful for the cooperation and warmth of the many patients, families, friends and neighbors who were patient with her questions. Bismillahi!

53

Sometimes I just get mad and cuss at them; call them sonsabitches. Sometimes that will work to make them be quiet for a while.

B.B., 79 years old, female, citizen of Tacoma, Washington

Both of these statements were made in response to being asked if there was anything, any task, that the respondents could perform that would silence what were called "sauti" (RA) or "extra-sensory perception communications" (BB). These phenomena are labelled "auditory hallucinations" in medical parlance and they are practically pathognomonic of schizophrenia, a diagnosis both respondents share. Both reported arguing, answering back and finally speaking profanity to be the only effective means for silencing the disembodied voices they hear. As an occupational therapist I would have been delighted to hear that engaging in some purposeful, playful or productive task helped keep the intrusive hallucinations at bay, but this was not the case.

Of these two women one is young, the other is old. One is black, one is white. One lives in a poor socialist country, the other in a rich capitalist country. One lives at home with her mother and her sister, the other in an institution with elderly people. For both of them the hallucinatory voices are generally cruel or critical, occasionally threatening or commanding. Sometimes they are the voices of women. More often they are the voices of men. Sometimes it is hard to tell anything about the owners of the voices. Both women take neuroleptics and in neither case is this sufficient to produce quiet for them. Although they report cursing the disembodied speakers of criticism, neither usually does so in a voice that is audible.

MADNESS, CULTURE, BIOLOGY AND ME

In Zanzibar, there are a number of Kiswahili words that can be employed to describe insanity. All cultures seem to have a word or words to label behavior that is deviant from the norm and that involves a disturbance not believed to be purely physical and or to be voluntary. Terms like "mental disorder," "mental illness," "psychosis," and "schizophrenia" have replaced "hysteria," "lunacy," "madness," "dementia praecox" and others in the history of Western medicine. Modern existential psychiatrists, like Szasz (1961) and Laing (1964), and feminists like Chesler (1972) have chosen to use the term "madness" in their critiques of the medical model of intervention in disturbed or disturbing behavior. Thus, in describing cross-cultural similarities and differences in what Western medicine labels "schizophrenia," I too have chosen to employ the term "madness."

I went to Africa because I wanted to observe madness in another cultural context. I had kept up with many of the recent developments in schizophrenia research: the refinements of the dopamine hypothesis, the computerized axial tomography findings of ventricular enlargement, the positron emission tomography findings of diminished frontal lobe activity, the documentation of neurological soft signs. I had come to see schizophrenia as a neurobiological disorder. Yet I knew that its expression was influenced by sociocultural forces. My interest in the neurobiology of schizophrenia lent more enthusiasm to my lectures on sensory integrative approaches to treatment of psychosis than I was able to muster for lectures on occupational behavior approaches. I wondered if occupational therapy theories on treatment of psychosocial dysfunction had validity in cultures other than that which spawned them. I needed time away from teaching to sort out my own thoughts and ideas about schizophrenia, its neurobiological nature, its sociocultural expression, its treatment.

Having been granted a one-year sabbatical leave from the University of Puget Sound, I procured a position with the Ministry of Health of Zanzibar, Tanzania. I had no sponsoring or sending agency. My Tanzanian salary was the equivalent of $40 per month. In exchange for designing an occupational therapy program for the 100 bed mental hospital at Kidongo Chekundu and training someone to run it after I was gone, I was given permission, encouragement and staff support to study schizophrenia in my own way.

ZANZIBAR AND SWAHILI CULTURE

It is often said that Zanzibar has too much history for so little geography. The two small islands in the Indian Ocean that comprise it, Unguja and Pemba, have been Portuguese, Omani Arab and

British possessions. Today, Zanzibar is a sovereign state within the United Republic of Tanzania. The population of the two islands is about 600,000 with nearly one quarter residing in Zanzibar town proper on Unguja (Garssen et al., 1989). The central city of very old stone buildings with carved wooden doors has winding streets that are only wide enough to allow for foot traffic and well maneuvered bicycles.

The Zanzibaris, like most coastal East Africans from southern Somalia to northern Mozambique, are Swahili people who share a common history, culture, language (Kiswahili) and religion (Islam). They are descendants of Africans who settled the coastal strip and islands in the 5th and 6th centuries and of traders who emigrated there to escape natural disasters, religious turmoil and civil wars in Persia and Arabia between the 7th and 10th centuries. The Zanzibari people are mostly Sunni Muslims of the Shafite school although there are small groups of other sects and schools (e.g., Ibadhi). Women wear black *bui bui* veils in public which cover their heads and their dresses but do not conceal their faces. For prayers men wear a *kanzu*, an ankle length shirt and a *kofia*, embroidered skull cap. Businesses and offices close at noon on Friday for prayers. In the old Stone Town area of Zanzibar town alone there are more than 30 mosques. Small Roman Catholic, Anglican Catholic and Hindu congregations also exist. Relations between Muslims and non-Muslims appear cordial, respectful and tolerant yet people very rarely marry outside their faith.

The extended family is the basic social unit with most leisure time spent in homosocial groupings within it. Care of children is shared between various generations and branches of a family. A child has many mothers and fathers, for the siblings of the biological parents share this title. Children live with other than their biological parents for extended periods of time, beginning at weaning. Grandparents and opposite sex grandchildren share a special relationship. The average age of marriage for women is 18.6 years. Women report wanting more than six children on average (Garssen, 1988). Traditionally marriage is arranged but adherence with this custom varies by family. The consent of the young woman is considered in the majority of cases and couple will have met and socialized before the arrangement is made. Polygamy is legal although at this time economics mitigate against its practice.

Cloves are the number one export crop. With clove prices falling and a cheaper, albeit inferior, product from Indonesia flooding the market, times are hard in Zanzibar. Fishing, agriculture and animal husbandry are both government enterprises and subsistence strategies for families. The government sector and small business employ many. Yet, there is much unemployment, especially among youth. It is more common than not to have more than one form of enterprise to sustain the family, and a man feels fortunate to have this situation. For example, one co-worker of mine had his government service job at the hospital, kept several cows and sold milk, cultivated cassava to sell in the market and burned coral to make lime.

THE HOSPITAL SETTING

Kidongo Chekundu Mental Hospital was built during the British era and is being refurbished by DANIDA, the Danish International Development Agency. Adequate potable water is available but must be carried at times as the pumping system is inadequate. The hospital stands in central eastern Zanzibar town just a 10 minute bus ride from the main market and old Stone Town. The neighborhood has concrete block, coral and lime, and traditional mud and thatch houses. The hospital, concrete block with red tile roofs, has 100 beds and runs at 60 to 70% capacity. Most of the patients come from the town. There are twice as many male patients as female. There are four wards, two for men and two for women; one of each is locked. Several wards have been closed, no longer in use. The furnishings are simple; disintegrating foam mattresses on rusting iron bed steads. Each ward has an open covered *baraza* where patients sit on the floor. Medication, provided in part through the DANIDA Essential Drugs Program, is distributed three times a day. The hospital is clean. Patients sweep and wash the wards daily, and some slash the grass and cultivate the cassava fields which surround the hospital. Yet there is insufficient organized work and inadequate numbers of tools for use in occupying the many idle hours for most patients.

Outpatients from the community line up at the dispensary each day where drugs and advice are dispensed and wounds are dressed. Malaria, diarrheal diseases, anemia and upper respiratory infections are the complaints most frequently treated at local dispensaries

(Garssen, 1989). Like most mental health services in Africa, Kidongo Chekundu is neuropsychiatric in its coverage; it cares for those with mental illnesses and epilepsy. It is the only facility for diagnosis and treatment of these disorders serving the 600,000 people of Zanzibar. Attempts are being made to provide better follow-up care at the islands' 74 dispensaries with the aim of decentralizing neuropsychiatric services.

Kidongo Chekundu is a relatively quiet peaceful place. The quiet is occasionally broken by the repetitive singing of one young man who is in the hospital as much as he is out. Rarely are patients restrained. Occasionally they are brought in tied with rope. School children walk through the hospital compound as they come and go for their studies for the place is neither walled nor fenced. Family members visit patients in the shade of the big tree in front of the nursing office perhaps bringing a special bit of food from home. Others bring male infants to the male nurses for circumcision, for the *Ukimwi* (AIDS) posters around town carry warnings about unclean implements in use by traditional practitioners. Little boys come to chase the pack of mangy homeless dogs that inhabit the hospital compound; dogs which everyone detests but no one has the inclination (or a good method) to kill.

HOSPITAL AND COMMUNITY RELATIONS

A patient on the roof trying to escape will bring out a crowd of the neighbors, young and old alike, to watch the action. Madness has entertainment value. The public soccer matches between teams of patients have been discontinued for it was felt that the laughter of the crowd was countertherapeutic. Madmen seem more pitied or ridiculed than feared or shunned.

Often one meets male patients, out on discharge or absconded, in the market place. One stands out because he is dirty and unshaven in a culture where cleanliness is highly valued. Another is seen eating bread on the street at high noon during the holy month of fasting, Ramadhan. Surely he must be mad. Another goes about with only short pants and no shirt, contravening adult male social norms of modesty and dress. And one sees old Yusuf, all cleaned up and freshly dressed each evening, out shopping and conversing with shop owners. He has lived at the hospital since his boyhood in the British colonial era and now has no family to go to. There is little wrong with him that institutional living did not cause. Even he, himself says, "You cannot put me out. I have no other home but Kidongo Chekundu now."

FROM OCCUPATIONAL THERAPY RESEARCH INTO THE WORLD OF SPIRITS

Although I had come to look at schizophrenia through the lenses of occupational therapy theories like sensory integration and human occupation, it soon became apparent that the unseen world of spirits was important to my understanding of the Swahili view of madness. I had planned to administer The Schroeder-Block-Campbell (SBC) Adult Psychiatric Sensory Integration Evaluation, the One Day Activity Chart and a devised set of culturally relevant functional skills items as a means to test the cross-cultural viability of different approaches to assessment. (A full report on that study is forthcoming.) I spent my first days at the hospital, sitting in the open air equivalent of the "day room" on each of the four wards, just watching, listening, and conversing. I had studied Kiswahili for 18 months before arriving. I wanted, first, only to immerse myself in the language, to get to know hospital routine and to look among the regular staff for someone to serve as my assistant and counterpart. Although I was moderately fluent in Kiswahili and had studied the history, literature, politics and economics of the region, I was ignorant of spirit beliefs and their relevance to madness.

On my first day on the locked men's ward a young teacher who had been brought to the hospital for flag desecration was teaching me how to play *bao*, an ancient counting game, with instruction in both Kiswahili and English. Another young man, Ali Bakar, smiling and talking much too fast for me to catch anything but "Sure, baby" and other interjections of English, sat beside me apparently to lend support and encouragement. He repeated something which drew frowns from some onlookers and smiles from others. The nurse who was subsequently to become my counterpart translated. Ali Bakar had invoked the aid of his *rohani*, a type of spirit, to ensure my victory in the game.

After this phase of ward observation, weeks were spent translating the test and interview schedules for my originally planned study and pilot testing the directions and questions with volunteers from the nursing staff and with student nurses. As my counterpart, Ahmed Awadh Salim, and I revised and became satisfied with the translations, I decided to test some in-patients with diagnoses other than schizophrenia as a final check of the translaton. Immediately again, the issue of the unseen world of spirits arose.

The first patient tested was a 40 year old woman with depression. She was from a rural community and, when asked to follow a demonstrated request that she hop on one foot (an SBC item for testing lateral dominance), told us that she could not comply because she had been bewitched, was made to feel heavy and had a *shetani*, a spirit causing this trouble. The next patient tested, a 15 year old girl from rural south Zanzibar had epilepsy. She said that she was unable to write with a pencil because the night before she had gotten a *shetani* who made it impossible for her to read and write. This explanation of *shetani* troubles was offered as the reason she could not add nor remember a common card game, abilities she reported she had once had, but lost.

In the course of our work on the assessment project it became clear that I needed to know what patients and their families thought about their problems and what meaning these "madnesses" had in the cultural context of Zanzibar. It became apparent that being mad or having a mad person in the family was a practical problem that required decisions about how to view the problem and where to turn for help. I added more questions to the interview schedule for the last 23 patients in the testing series already in progress. While those interviews were being conducted on a daily basis, I sought other avenues for learning about the Zanzibari view of madness, the spirit world, the curative use of the Koran and other forms of traditional treatment. I arranged for Ahmed to interview two patients with schizophrenia and their families in depth over several sessions. In those interviews we followed Spradley's (1979) guidelines for ethnographic interview. We also interviewed an 89 year old woman who was recognized for her knowledge of traditional beliefs related to madness. Less formal interviews were conducted with friends, neighbors and acquaintances. What a people value and what they believed about madness will affect their practices and attitudes related to it. This is true here in the U.S. and in Zanzibar. The interview project taught me some important things about how beliefs about madness affect the role and treatment of the mad person in the community. Such observations can be instructive for those practicing in the mental health field here and abroad.

CAUSATION BELIEFS

Lambo (1980) emphasized the necessity of examining perceptions of both the immediate and remote causes of disease in traditional belief systems. Edgerton (1966) and Neki et al. (1986) expressed similar ideas saying that the clinician or researcher must ask both "*How* did the illness come about?" and "*Why* did it come about?" The Swahili of Zanzibar believe that madness may be caused by spirit possession, witchcraft and sorcery and may be treated successfully with traditional Koran based treatments. Neki and his colleagues, based on experience with Swahili and other Bantu peoples in Dar-es-Salaam, Tanzania, pointed out that witchcraft as a theory of causation "does not deny natural or empirical causes but seeks supernatural causes behind them" (Neki et al., 1986, pg. 146). They saw witchcraft beliefs so common among their patients at Muhimbili Medical Center that they found it useful to delineate differences in delusional witchcraft beliefs and ordinary witchcraft beliefs and to elaborate strategies for dealing with them in psychotherapy.

Many of the schizophrenic patients interviewed believed that they presently had or at one time had a *shetani* that accounted for the symptoms of what we labelled schizophrenia. A *shetani* may be picked up accidentally or it may be sent through witchcraft. The two non-schizophrenic patients described above both claimed to have *mashetani* (the plural) via bewitchment. *Mashetani* possess the afflicted, take control and cause her to act in ways she would not ordinarily. It is widely held that everyone has *ashetani*; this is considered customary and natural. Problems come when one's *shetani* is disgruntled or angry or when one is occupied by an additional malintentioned *shetani*.

There are a variety of ways one might get an additional *shetani*.

One can inherit a *shetani* from the recently deceased or someone may send one to another person. *Mashetani* may be trapped in bottles and buried or released upon someone. Burying a *shetani*-containing vessel or releasing a bottled *shetani* near someone are ways to cause that person harm. This is *uchawi* (witchcraft), as is petitioning a witch to send a shetani to someone. The situation of being away from home, particularly on the road, seems to carry some additional risk of troublesome *shetani* occupation. In one case, for example, a patient's mother thought her daughter's trip to the mainland to college precipitated her problems because of picking up a *shetani* along the way. Another interpretation in the same case was that a jealous co-worker had sent it. One might risk occupation by a *shetani* by loitering in places where *mashetani* are said to live such as baobab trees, big mango trees and in ruined or abandoned buildings.

Mashetani are not seen as necessarily evil by their nature. Accounts of useful or helpful *mashetani* are rare but some people are said to cultivate them as allies or even to keep them as pets. Rather than good or evil, *mashetani* are seen as changeable and thus, always potentially troublesome. They do not wish to be ignored or forgotten. If things are going well one must not forget to acknowledge the *shetani* and offer it a bit of coffee or other treat. If angered, *mashetani* can cause a variety of troubles including seizures and madness. A troublesome *shetani* may make one quiet and withdrawn or loud, voluble and erratic. They can make one sick, although not necessarily with some named disease. One simply will not feel well. The afflicted may feel weak and lethargic and his head will most certainly ache and feel heavy.

One can apply the dichotomies immediate/remote causes, as suggested by Lambo (1980), and how/why of causation to *shetani* and witchcraft beliefs is the Zanzibari belief system. Witchcraft was seen by Neki (1986) as the answer to the "why." If witchcraft is the "why" then the troublesome shetani is the "how." Yet both seem more immediate than remote. One thing is certain: in Zanzibar the remote but ultimate cause was always given as the will of Allah, often expressed as *shauri ya Mungu* (plan or intention of God) or as *rehema ya Mungu* (mercy or wish of God). When asked why someone might want to harm a child (necessitating the wearing of amulets for protection) an 89 year old woman merely replied *"kiduniani"* or "the way of the world." Thus either divine or human agents may cause one harm for unknown reasons.

Supernatural causes for madness were not the only ones elicited in our interviews. More mundane causes included smoking marijuana, drinking alcohol and studying too hard. Most respondents were also aware that cerebral malaria could produce agitated, deranged behavior. Mundane and supernatural causes are seen to interact in the production of disturbed behavior. A jealous rival may send one a *shetani* via witchcraft while studying for a big examination. One may offend Allah by consuming alcohol and be allowed to contract malarial fever.

CURATIVE PRACTICES

Respondents differentiated "European" sicknesses, for which "hospital" medicine was appropriate, from "local" sicknesses for which traditional Swahili medicine was appropriate. When madness was ascribed to a *shetani* whether acquired via witchcraft or accident, traditional treatment was chosen. Certain traditional treatments may be performed by family members, usually females. More elaborate ones require a *sheik* who can read and write Koranic verse or an *mganga*, a traditional healer who may use exorcism, botanical and/or Koran based remedies. Such specialists exact a price for services, however.

Subjects who had schizophrenia and their families reported resort to both traditional medicine and to hospital medicine for different episodes of similar behavior depending upon how the behavior was labelled. The label *shetani* appeared no more stable over time than other labels for madness; that is, episodes of very similar behavior might be attributed to a *shetani* at one time or given some other label at another time. Sometimes the presence of a *shetani* was only confirmed after successful traditional treatment. Madness tends to be recurring and it may remit spontaneously. Thus, many families with a member who had schizophrenia were called upon to choose between coexisting treatment systems on more than one occasion when either or both systems were perceived as effective to some extent. In about 60% of the cases we studied, traditional treatment had been sought first and then a change was made to reliance on hospital (or clinic) treatment. In 35% of the cases change was bidirectional: beginning with traditional treatment, changing to hospital treatment, back to traditional treatment and back to hospital treatment again. In only 5% of cases did treatment choice begin with the hospital, change to traditional treatment and back to hospital treatment again. It is important to note that all of the reports end with hospital treatment only because we were interviewing hospital patients and their families. In a random sample of the Zanzibari population selected for an epidemiological survey only 14% of those identified with mental disorders never sought traditional treatment (Garssen et al., 1989). An equal number always sought traditional treatment. The remaining majority resorted to both systems. It is not at all the case that hospital treatment of disturbed behavior was perceived as better or more effective. One elderly female patient told us that she preferred traditional treatment, stating "If you go to the *mganga* you will see many different medicines, roots, grasses and the like, but here you have just one thing, white pills, but they are free." Cost was one of the major factors considered in choosing between the coexisting systems for treating madness. The effects of cost and of other factors on decision making are summarized in Table 1.

VALUES AND ATTITUDES REGARDING MADNESS, ITS CAUSES AND CURES

Cultural values and childrearing practices contribute to a strong sense in the Swahili person of being a member of a cohesive group. The authority of elders is viewed as natural and is not easily questioned. The group and its well being are valued over individual freedom and identity. Identity is derived more from the family than from individual accomplishments. Cooperation is valued over competition. Witchcraft beliefs are consistent with the value placed on cooperation and the importance of the group over that of the individual. Standing out as an individual causes jealousy which can make one vulnerable to ill will. It is better to blend in harmoniously and to work for the good of the group. *Mchezo kwao hutunzwa*

Table 1. **Determinants of resort to hospital or traditional treatment in cases labelled schizophrenic on hospitalization**

Hospital treatment selected if:
Home administered traditional treatments failed
Healer administered treatment failed to change behavior, or relapse occurred
There was no money to pay for traditional treatment (hospital is free)
Patient could not be subdued for transport to a traditional healer
Patient had come into police custody
Patient was feverish and malaria was suspected
Decision was in the hands of a male family member with secondary education
Previous hospital treatment was perceived as successful

Traditional treatment selected if:
Hospital treatment failed to change behavior, or relapse occurred
Someone in the family had a botanical remedy available
Someone in the family could read Koran
There was money available to pay a healer outside the family
There was reason to believe others were jealous of or angry with the patient
Decision was in the hands of a female family member with limited education
Previous traditional treatment was perceived as successful

states the proverb: he who puts his efforts in his collectively shared place is rewarded.

Problems and troubles are expected in human life. "After all," the Swahili people say, "this is not heaven, this is only the world." When pressed to make a value judgment about her daughter's sickness, one mother's response captures much of the acquiescence of the Swahili world view: "Each one knows his own burden best. . . . I can not say if this sickness is a bad thing worse than others. God may give his blessings to somebody, I do not know the reasons. Allah will not send more than we can bear." The impermanence of the *shetani* label, the belief that everyone has a shetani which may become troublesome, the cohesiveness of the family and the belief that the ultimate cause for madness is Allah's wishes seemed to support family acceptance of persons labelled schizophrenic. In only a very few cases were patients detained at the hospital longer than considered necessary by lack of a placement for them. I recall that one young woman was detained longer than usual because her grandfather wanted more time for his neighbors to forget and forgive. During a psychotic episode the young woman had destroyed a cassava field and with it a portion of the neighbors' livelihood. This example stands out because patients were generally accepted back into their families of origin, nuclear or extended, with little hesitation. They were given tasks to perform according to their abilities and gender roles as before.

It is unclear from our data and from that of the 1988 epidemiology study what the measurable impact of madness is on social status (Garssen et al., 1989). In the probability sample obtained for the epidemiological study most Zanzibari women over the age of 30 who had a mental disorder were separated or divorced, but all had been married. Only 17% of males identified in the same survey as having mental disorders were separated or divorced but an additional 50% had never married. Marriage is nearly universal and only 2.5% of Zanzibari women remain childless (Garssen, 1988). In our sample of 17 hospital treated schizophrenics, only one man lived with his wife, three women with their husbands and the remaining majority of respondents lived with other family members. Marriage is openly acknowledged in traditional Swahili culture to be primarily an economic arrangement with the Western concept of romantic love playing a very small role. None of our interview sample of 17 individuals with schizophrenia reported living alone nor did any of the 23 mentally ill individuals identified in the epidemiological survey (Garssen et al., 1989). Group homes, boarding homes and similar institutions do not exist in Zanzibar. Thus mentally ill people live at the hospital or at home with family.

COMPARISONS AND CONTRASTS

I have not yet undertaken a systematic series of ethnographic interviews with Americans with schizophrenia and their families. Yet I have practiced in psychiatric institutions, served on a mental health advisory board with the parents of people with schizophrenia, and currently treat a woman with schizophrenia. Further, I have a good friend whose son is diagnosed with schizophrenia and I have spent many hours in conversation with my friend soliciting his beliefs about the problem. Drawing from these experiences, I will examine the interplay of American beliefs, values and attitudes toward schizophrenia to compare it with what I observed in Zanzibar. It may be easier for us to see how "exotic" elements of a foreign culture affect what is believed and done about a problem like madness. Yet, the dominant culture of twentieth century America affects what we believe and do about schizophrenia here in very much the same way that Swahili culture shapes beliefs and practices related to madness there.

Sanchez (1964), writing about the potential effects of cultural values on occupational therapy, summarized the often unquestioned cultural values of the American middle and upper classes as emphasizing: (1) the individual over the group, (2) the future over the present, (3) control of nature or fate by exertion of human will and power, (4) the importance of doing over that of being and (5) a view of human nature as perfectible. To Sanchez' list, I would add: (6) a tendency toward explanation of natural phenomena by reductionistic causality, (7) a belief in a mind/body dichotomy with the mind as the entity of control and (8) valuing science and rationality over religion and spirituality. Many American beliefs, practices and attitudes about schizophrenia can be understood in light of these eight cultural values.

Ask an American what causes mental illness, in general, or schizophrenia, in particular and you are likely to hear about bad genes or chemical imbalances. We have much more to say about the "how" of causation than the "why"; our beliefs about mental illness deal more with immediate than remote causes. I know two ministers with offspring with schizophrenia. Neither has ever expressed to me that the illness was in any way related to supernatural activity.

We consider schizophrenia an illness, a disease or a disorder. Although we can cite genetic inheritance as a predisposing cause and we may know of neurological abnormalities commonly found in schizophrenia, we call it a "mental" illness, not a neurological disorder or brain disease. We say it is not curable but manageable. We are looking for a "cure." Our label "schizophrenia" is considered permanent. The Diagnostic and Statistical Manual of the American Psychiatric Association, Third edition, Revised has a category for individuals with schizophrenia who are no longer schizo-phrenic (American Psychiatric Association, 1987). We health pro-fessionals may feel it our responsibility to convince people with schizophrenia that they will always have this disorder so that they will remain compliant with taking medication.

In talking about looking for a cure, families of American schizo-phrenics often express hope that the right combination of medica-tions can be found. They are often aware of the negative effects of psychopharmaceutical treatment as well. Belief in bimolecular cau-sality is consistent with belief in bimolecular treatment. While there is good evidence that monozygotic twins have high concordance rates for schizophrenia and that dopamine receptor blocking drugs diminish some symptoms in many of those we call schizophrenic, I do not believe that we know with any more certainty than the aver-age Zanzibari what causes some people to hear disembodied voices, for example, and others not to. Considering a hierarchy of explana-tion levels from sociocultural to interpersonal to intrapersonal to physiological to biochemical and on down to particle physics we seem, as a culture inclined to imbue the lower more reductionistic levels with more explanatory power than more holistic levels are given (Rose, 1976). Correlation is mistaken for causation and the more reductionistic of two phenomena believed to explain the other. Bad genes and chemical imbalances are assumed to account for odd behavior and not vice versa.

Other hopes are expressed as the wish that the family member with schizophrenia will "learn" something (like not to listen to the commanding voices), "understand" something, "develop in-sight," "master" some impulse, "achieve some discipline," "show some initiative." These hopes reflect the belief that learning or unlearning can change behavior, that the mind controls the body and that the person with schizophrenia is the most important actor on his own behalf capable of exerting his power or will to change the situation. The activity he is expected to undertake is described in mentalistic terms.

Families of Americans with schizophrenia express frustration, sometimes to the point of rage, despair, disappointment, and hurt when talking about their experiences with the disease they see as "the enemy." Frustration is often related to loss of perceived con-trol. The son or daughter's reaching the age of majority when parents no longer control treatment decisions or financial arrangements can be a crisis point for the family. One mother related stories of having to bar her daughter from the house so that she would meet the criteria for commitment and get services against her will. Had the family extended food and shelter to her she would not be considered at high enough risk for intervention by the state. One parent reported feeling "powerless to protect" his son. Despair seems linked to the perceived permanence of the disease and the limited ability of current treatments to eradicate symptoms. Americans express disappointment by emphasizing what a beautiful, charismatic or promising child the patient was before the illness. They are hurt by the lack of caring reciprocity or affection from this person who has changed, often "beyond recognition." Swahili people are, perhaps, protected from this hurt when ascribing changed behavior by a now unrecognizable family member to an invading spirit.

We are individuals with a free will, who can and should achieve independence and autonomy through mastery of the environment. We are each on an individual trajectory into the future. We are healthy and good when our "locus of control" is internal (Rotter 1966; Oakley, Kielhofner and Barris, 1985). We have the ability to be masters of our own destinies to a great extent. If we want something enough and are willing to work for it, we can get it. We are to be sociable, of course, but not lose our individual identity. We are each unique.

The paragraph above is not a series of statements of natural fact. It is what the dominant culture shapes us to believe. These beliefs would seem as odd to a traditional Swahili person as belief in *shetani* possession is to readers of this essay. The American legal system and social structure are founded on the absolute value of individual rights. It is important to note that families sometimes perceive these institutions as interfering with their expressions of concern for mentally ill family members. Our view of ourselves and others is shaped by our valuing of individuality, of the future and of control over nature through exertion of human will. The concepts of personal causation, temporal adaptation, valued goals and personal interests as described in the occupational therapy literature are shaped by these same dominant culture values (Neville, 1980; Barris, Kielhofner and Watts, 1983).

CONCLUSION

Madness or psychosis is a complex alteration of perceived reality which manifests itself with certain similarities cross-culturally (Murphy, 1976). It is neurobiological, psychosocial and sociocultural in expression and in its impact. Its causes seem to be multifactorial. It is not my intention here to show that one set of values or beliefs, one culture or the other, is better or to advocate that Americans adopt the values and beliefs of the Zanzibari Swahili. That would be foolish and futile. Rather, I would have us recognize the relativity of our beliefs and values, and the context in which we have adopted them so that we might examine their effects on our attitudes and practices as health care professionals. Not all American subscribe to the values and beliefs of the dominant culture. If we unquestioningly assume that they do when we devise our theoretical models or design treatment, we risk disrespecting and discounting the legitimacy of other humans' world views. Treatment will fail. Models of human occupation ought to be applicable to all humans. As the African psychiatrist Lambo (1980, pg 370) wrote, "In the African world, reality is found in the soul, in religious acquiescence to life, not in its mastery. Reality rests on the relations between one human being and another, and between all people and spirits."

REFERENCES

American Psychiatric Association. (1987). *Diagnostic and statistical manual of mental disorders*. Third Edition, revised. Washington, D.C.: American Psychiatric Association.

Barris, R., Kielhofner, G., & Watts, J. (1983). *Psychosocial occupational therapy: practice in a pluralistic arena*. Laurel, MD: RAMSCO.

Chesler, P. (1972). *Women and madness*. New York, NY: Doubleday.

Edgerton, R.B. (1966). Conceptions of Psychosis in Four East African Societies. *American Anthropologist. 68*, 408-425.

Garssen, J. (1988). *Mortality, fertility and contraceptive knowledge, attitudes and practices in Zanzibar: Results of the 1988 survey*. Zanzibar, Tanzania: Ministry of Health.

Garsen, J. Haji, H.M. (1989). *Statistical tables for health planners*. Health Information Bulletin No. 47, Zanzibar, Tanzania: Ministry of Health.

Garssen, J., Abdulwakil, A.I., Bondestam, S. (1989). *The mental health pro-*

gramme in Zanzibar: Results of the 1988 Survey on prevalence and treatment of mental disorders and epilepsy. Zanzibar, Tanzania: Ministry of Health.

Laing, R.D. & Esterson, A. (1964). *Sanity, madness and the family.* New York: Basic Books.

Lambo, T.A. (1980). Psychotherapy in Africa. *In Conformity and Conflict.* New York, NY: Little, Brown & Co.

Neki, J.S., Joinet, B., Ndosi, N., Kilonzo, G., Hauli, J.G., & Duvinage, G. (1986). Witchcraft and psychotherapy. *British Journal of Psychiatry. 149,* 145-155.

Murphy, J.M. (1976). Psychiatric labelling in cross cultural perspective. *Science. 191,* 1019-1028.

Neville, A (1980). Temporal adaptation: Application with short-term psychiatric patients. *American Journal of Occupational Therapy. 34,* 328-331.

Oakley, F., Kielhofner, G., and Barris, R. (1985). An occupational therapy approach to assessing psychiatric patients' adaptive functioning. *American Journal of Occupational Therapy. 39,* 147-154.

Rose, S (1976). *The conscious brain.* New York: Random House.

Rotter, J. (1966). Generalized expectancies of internal versus external control of reinforcement. *Psychological Monographs: General Applied. 80,* 1-28.

Sanchez, V. (1964). Relevance of cultural values for occupational therapy programs. *American Journal of Occupational Therapy. 18,* 1-5.

Schroeder, C.V., Block, M.P., Trottier, E.C. & Stowell, M.S. (1978). *Schroeder, Block, Campbell, adult psychiatric sensory integration battery.* Second experimental edition. La Jolla, CA: SBC Research Associates.

Spradley, J. (1979). *The ethnographic interview.* New York: Holt, Rinehart, Winston.

Szasz, T.S. (1961). *The myth of mental illness: Foundations of a theory of personal conduct.* New York: Hoeber-Harper.

Evaluating the Developmental Skills
of Cambodian Orphans

Lynn Miller, OTR, RPT, MEd

SUMMARY. The author found the experience of evaluating orphans in Cambodia different from her expectations and it has changed her attitudes toward education and medicine. She suggests that all prospective orphans be evaluated by a therapist in order to anticipate the severity of potential problems. She also feels that occupational therapists must take an active role in affecting the lives of people in third world countries. The author discusses how her experience is shaping her professional goals since she returned from Cambodia.

I could not have been happier. I was surrounded by children, more children than I could possibly ever evaluate. I did not need to read any files for there were none. I did not have to get parent permissions to test, for their parents had been killed by the Cambodians' relentless war over the last 25 years. I could just sit all day on the tile floor, for there were no tables or chairs, and evaluate one child at a time. I had come to Cambodia with a small group of prospective parents from World Family Hawaii Adoption Agency, after having convinced its director, Dr. Daniel Sussot, that he could use my services in evaluating the physical abilities of the children he hoped to adopt.

I had been to Cambodia once before when I had worked my way around the world in 1964. Then Phnom Penh was the Paris of the east with wide boulevards full of flowering trees, elegant restaurants and European-type Hotels. This was before the Vietnam war

Lynn Miller has worked in Denmark and Japan, taught in the OT Department at the University of New Hampshire and now works in the public schools in the United States. Her address is 9 Orchard Drive, Durham, NH 03824.

and before all the massive bombing they received from the United States. This was before the Khymer Rouge took over in 1978 and mercilessly tortured and killed a million of their own population. Those of us who have seen the movie "The Killing Fields" can picture some of the horrors. The last ten years with the Vietnamese in control has actually just continued the civil war. Presently there are four factors vying for control, with military and arms support coming from China, the Soviet Union and the United States. The United Nations continues to try to initiate peace talks, but these efforts have yet to make much difference in the daily lives of the Cambodians.

Our daily lives were difficult too and at times the problems seemed almost insurmountable. Besides the inefficient communist bureaucracy, we had to make arrangements for adopting the children in Phnom Penh, where there were no phones, no radios, no newspapers, few cars, no computers, little electricity, no streetlights, and an enforced curfew after nine o'clock. Government officials changed frequently and only a few could speak any language besides Khymer, for all the educated people were killed by the Khymer Rouge. Recent fighting outside the city made us feel trapped inside its limits and explosions going off occasionally in the streets made us nervous. We even had preplanned escape routes which we fortunately did not need to use.

THE CHILDREN

So there I was, doing what I do best and loving every minute. I could observe, think and describe the characteristics of the child I saw before me. Even the hundred degree heat did not dampen my enthusiasm. And although I have worked with children for the past 15 years, babies as well as school age kids, I did not expect what I found.

In a third world country, without much modern technology, nor medicine, I expected to find many severely handicapped children. I thought I would find many children who suffered difficulties at birth and might be brain damaged, since there would obviously be no intensive care units in their hospitals. I anticipated I would find children who had meningitis, or spina bifida, and other neurological conditions that are difficult to treat. All the international articles from Occupational Therapy and Physical Therapy newspapers mentioned treating children with cerebral palsy; adapting chairs and crutches for them.

What I found was that most of the children were doing surprisingly well and especially at first glance seemed extremely normal. In spite of severely deprived lives, little food, no medicine, and not much adult attention, they seemed incredibly healthy. Most were physically active, intellectually curious, and appropriately trusting. I did not find one low tone, fragile looking four year old at the orphanage. Almost all of these children could run, jump, catch and kick balls, and manipulate tiny items with their hands.

There were however a few children who were not doing as well. Several rooms of cribs had tiny babies lying on their backs, with weak, pathetic little cries, fighting for their lives. It was only too apparent that any child with any unusual complications just did not survive these early days. I felt I was stepping into a time predating the advent of modern medicine and was seeing only children who were able to live in spite of war, malnutrition, disease and the loss of their parents.

There were also some two and three year olds that were not developing well. Several looked malnourished and sat immobile on the floor, balancing themselves with their distended stomachs. They stared vacantly at me as I tried to interest them in my various toys. Since they spent most of their days in wooden cribs and were placed on the floor to play only a few hours each day, it was not surprising many did not walk until they were three years old (Picture 1). Some had polio and their joints were contracted in abnormal positions. I knew that some would never walk, and would probably never have crutches or wheelchairs. I tried to assess their developmental levels, but there was no way of knowing accurately the mental and physical abilities of these very sick young children. Supposedly many do well when adopted, but I had my own fears that even medicine, food and love were not going to be enough for some of these babies.

As I tested the four year old children, I became more and more aware of their poor expressive language. Here I was finding adorable bright children with beautiful eyes who could speak only a few

PHOTO 1. The two and three year olds were placed on the floor to play a few hours each day. Several of these children probably have had polio.

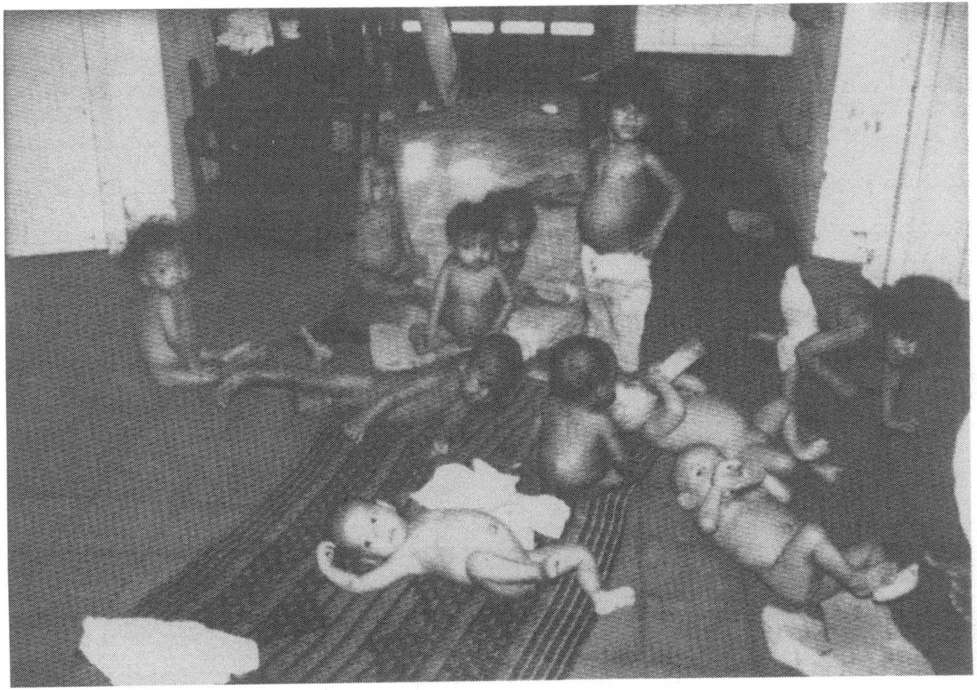

words. They supposedly understood everything, but said nothing, according to their caretaker. I worried about critical periods for language, neurological pathways, and being learning disabled for life. Would each adopted child be labelled speech and language delayed? Fortunately, I later found out that I need not have been so concerned, for the children learn their adoptive language quickly as their first language, not their second (Picture 2). It seems they have neither heard much language nor have they much reason to speak. They can understand the few sentences shouted at them "dinner time," "stop fighting," "time to go in." However they have heard sounds, they do make a wide variety of noises, and they do understand the usefulness of language.

New children arrived daily at the orphanage. One two month old baby we succeeded in adopting had been on a train the week before with her mother when the train was ambushed by the Khymer Rouge. Her mother was killed along with fifty others. Her father had died a hundred days before and her mother was returning from a special funeral service for him. The baby was brought in by a young couple who had been holding her when her mother went to get some fresh air at the doorway where she was shot.

I watched young twins brought in one time by a grandmother, saying that her daughter had died and she no longer could feed them. She held one in each arm. Both looked malnourished, with bloated stomachs and underdeveloped arms and legs. They were nearly two years of age, even though they looked more like six months.

I was struck by the fact that eighty percent of the children in the orphanage were boys. I found several reasons why this was the case. In Cambodian culture, girls are considered easier to raise, less demanding, less active, and therefore they are not given up for adoption as often. They also can be more useful at home, and tragically may be made to make a living at prostitution at a young age. Girls are also more desirable to adopt and so the few girls that do come to the orphanage are placed in new homes quickly. Boys on the other hand tend to be very active, and are given up for adoption more often, as well as tend to stay in the orphanage longer.

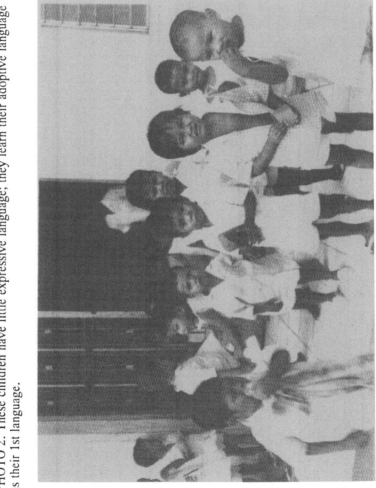

PHOTO 2. These children have little expressive language; they learn their adoptive language as their 1st language.

ASSESSMENT

I came equipped to use the standardized tests I usually use, "Birth to Three," and "Peabody Test for Motor Development." I even translated important sentences into French as I knew some of the caretakers could speak it. However, I knew right away that these assessments would be no more valid for the orphans than they are for neurologically involved children in the United States although for very different reasons (Photo 3). None of them had any of the background experiences that would lead to developing some of the skills on the lists.

These children, it seems, spend most of their time, either inside their rooms, which contain only cots and no toys, or outside their building running around on the grass, again without toys. They share an adult with twenty other children, and while these caretakers seemed pleasant, they can barely manage their little ones physically, let alone stimulate them mentally. These children knew no songs, had never seen a stacking toy, nor a puzzle, and rarely had a ball in their hands.

The children were herded as a group from one building to another to eat or to play and they were strictly controlled (Photo 4). It did become easier to understand why they had so little expressive language after watching their daily routine.

It is therefore no wonder that the children responded with unbridled enthusiasm to me, not only because they all craved affection, but I brought all the typical toys of an itinerant therapist (balls, tops, Rubik's cube, blocks, markers, wind up toys, gymnastic balls, balloons). I developed an alternative questionnaire and format, with my goal being to describe the present level of each child in a way that a prospective parent could easily understand some of the child's major characteristics. I divided the areas of interest into four main groups . . . Physical Characteristics, Personality, Intelligence and Caretaker Information. (See Table 1 at the end of the article.)

I worked with one child at a time, sharing my toys, trying to get him to feel comfortable with me. I looked at his response to the toys, his behavior, his skills, as well as analyzed the quality of his interaction and his movement. The more children I worked with, the easier it became to separate what seemed normal and age appro-

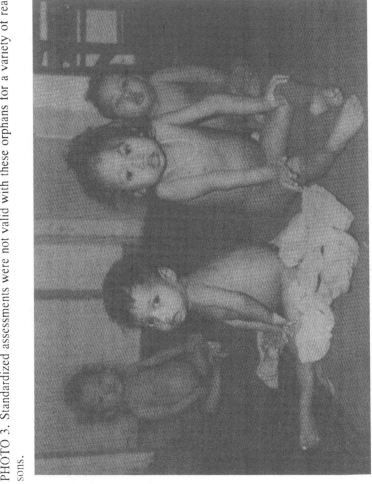

PHOTO 3. Standardized assessments were not valid with these orphans for a variety of reasons.

PHOTO 4. Most of these orphans have only minor medical problems and may have been adopted by now.

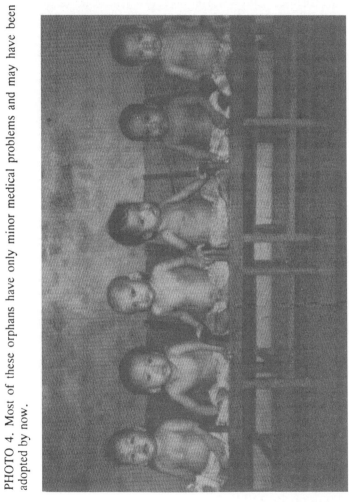

priate from what seemed unusual. I had to keep in mind that all Cambodian children look younger and are much smaller than I might think from their chronological age. I also used everything I knew as well as all I could sense or feel to bring out their abilities. It was both exhausting and exhilarating at the same time.

In spite of all their background differences, children are still children, and the orphans were no exception. They laughed and giggled, grabbed toys, and chased one another. They cried, they hugged, they piled on top of one another and me in an attempt to get physical contact. They moved their bodies in smooth coordinated ways, their eyes sparkled with humor, they showed kindness and understanding toward one another. They invented new ways to use a toy and remembered details about it. They showed a great deal about themselves in a short period of time, not the least was their ability to trust and be open to a stranger who could not speak any of their language, a most valuable skill for a prospective adoptee. My background in normal and abnormal development and in NDT allowed me to observe and judge quickly each child's areas of competence.

We were able to bring four children to the United States this last July and others I evaluated came out later in the fall. I made a follow-up visit to Maine in November to see one of the babies. She was developing well, giving me more hope and optimism about her future. The Adoption Agency is continuing its efforts because its enthusiastic and charismatic leader, Dr. Sussot, having worked for years as a doctor in the Cambodian refugee camps will never give up trying to help this once beautiful country.

PERSONAL AND PROFESSIONAL REFLECTIONS

Being in a third world country that is overcrowded and dysfunctional in so many ways makes me feel I have seen a glimpse of the future of our world; a world with too many people, families without homes, children without clothes, women without birth control, men without work, and disease, hunger and death becoming common human experiences.

I returned to the United States a different person. I now appreciate certain aspects of my life that I previously took for granted. I realized when I was in Cambodia that I have already lived longer than the average life expectancy there, even though I am still in my forties. I have also been able to control the number of children I have had and to expect that none would die. I have never had to worry about feeding them, nor have I ever gone hungry myself. I have never had a serious disease, nor even chronic infection or pain. I even have all my teeth. I have never lost a member of my family to war, nor do I have recurring nightmares of watching my parents or children raped or tortured. I appreciate the resiliency of the human spirit, now more than ever.

But professionally I am left in a dilemma, for nothing I do seems as important anymore. The size and number of the world's problems overwhelm me when I think about them, for half the world lives in a similar situation to Cambodia. We seem to act in the United States as if we have limitless resources and wealth, and can afford to take care of everyone as long as there is a breath of life. Our priorities seem all mixed up. How can we really justify spending hundreds of thousands of dollars on the severely brain injured with no potential for change when normal children die for lack of care? How can twelve professionals, including me, help mainstream one handicapped child in school, when large populations of our children become drop outs? What will our lives be like in ten or fifteen years when the hundreds of thousands or even millions of street children all over the world grow up without education or jobs? What would the cost be to inoculate all the children in Cambodia against polio? Similar to a bomber or to one day in Saudi Arabia? Why can't we spend money on prevention rather than waiting for the inevitable crisis?

My priorities as a therapist are shifting, but have not yet settled into a new pattern for me. I feel occupational therapists have incredibly useful skills to offer the world, in all of our specialties. I, probably, for example know more about the needs and the development of children than any one in all of Cambodia. I could improve the lives of the entire orphanage in a very substantial manner. But I spend my time with a much smaller number of children who have much less potential. Time seems to be more valuable and how we spend it seems more critical than ever. I find myself wanting to be involved with the care, treatment or even prevention of more serious problems. I want to make more of a difference for a larger number of children who have the possibility of living more fulfilled lives.

I feel I have become an even stronger occupational therapist. My interest in helping people, adults or children, obtain the highest quality of life possible for them becomes even stronger. But I become even more concerned that we must become involved in the prevention of some of the world's medical problems.

None of these issues is new, but the disparity between medical care here and in the third world countries has never been as great. Perhaps my own anguish will dissipate and I can again fit into our technological world, although I believe that there are two issues that seem somewhat approachable. I would appreciate any suggestions.

Polio, from a therapist's point of view, seems like the ultimate in preventable tragedies. I would like to become involved in reducing the number of cases, rather than only becoming efficient in treating them. The vaccine I know is particularly difficult to bring into countries with poor transportation, but there must be a way.

Secondly, I feel that all infants and children who are to be adopted in this country should be evaluated first by an expert in development, such as a pediatric occupational therapist. This way parents will not adopt children with problems beyond their abilities to manage (Picture 5). This would mean there may be many more therapists who would have third world experiences like mine. Perhaps our Occupational therapy curricula should include classes on cross cultural differences, on ways to work internationally and on our obligation to become more involved in world problems as a profession. Perhaps then together we can really make a difference.

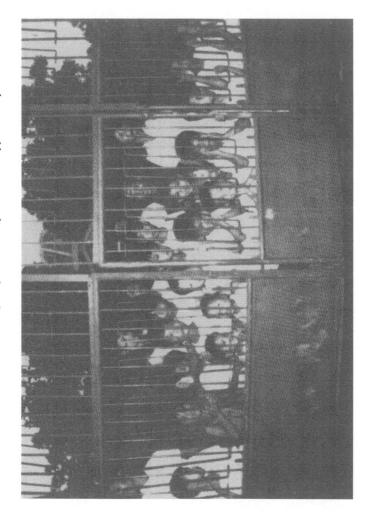

PHOTO 5. There are so many ways that occupational therapy can help others.

TABLE 1

ORPHAN CHECKLIST

Name _____

Sex

Age child appears

Date of Birth _____

Age

Date arrival at orphanage

Personality

Outgoing/Shy?
Affectionate?
Fearful/Cautious?
Cries a lot?
Smiles a lot?
Activity level?
Sense of humor?
Courage to try new activities?
Easy to play with:

Intelligence

Response time
Initiation of new method
Learned new toy quickly?
Age level interest in toys?
Curiosity?
Drawing? Draw-a-person

Physical Characteristic

Appearance?
Basic motor development
 - large motor -- age level?
 - good at?
 - fine motor -- pencil grip?
Basic health?
Condition of teeth?
Any asymmetries -- eyes?
    body?

Caretakers Comments

Health background
Behavior
Speech & language
 - receptive
 - expressive
Personality
Other special characteristics

Evaluator's Summary

Basic quality of interaction?
Most engaging characteristic?

Training in a Foreign Land
That is Home

Kristine Markewitz, OTR/L

SUMMARY. The author describes her pediatric Level II fieldwork experience in Southeast Alaska. She discusses her professional development during this time, and some of the differences between practice in Southeast Alaska and Seattle, Washington.

It was just over two years ago, in February of 1989, that I found myself boarding a ferry boat in my home port of Seattle, Washington, bound for Sitka, a small town in Southeast Alaska. It was a four day journey in the middle of winter and the beginning of my third and last Fieldwork Level II experience. As we rode along the coast of Canada and then up to the coast of Alaska the landscape became more and more rugged. In Canada the coastline was hilly and full of evergreens, similar to Washington, except that it appeared completely undeveloped. Alaska also appeared undeveloped, and was even more rugged. Sharp snow-drenched peaks began to emerge off the Alaskan coastline. It all appeared larger than anything I had ever seen; the wilderness stretched up and out as far as my eyes could see. Indeed there were rarely signs of human life

Kristine Markewitz studied occupational therapy at the University of Washington. Since completing her fieldwork in Alaska she has worked at Childhaven (a therapeutic daycare center for children at risk for abuse and neglect, and/or for children suffering from drug effects), at Overlake Hospital (on call, inpatient psychiatry), and at the Northshore School District. She currently works part-time at Childhaven and the Northshore School District. Her address is 506 17th Avenue East, Apartment 2, Seattle, WA 98112.

The author would like to acknowledge the faculty at the University of Washington, in particular Susie Cunningham, the coordinator of the rural pediatric training project, and also Mo McBride in Sitka, AK.

89

or activity for those first two days at sea, although there were signs of wildlife. We saw schools of porpoises in the water, deer feeding on the beaches, and sea birds everywhere.

On the third day of our voyage I realized just how foreign it all felt. That was when we made our first stop, in the small town of Wrangell, Alaska. I disembarked to view some petroglyphs on the beach. Then, while walking up an icy street, I saw a sign and was surprised to see that the words were in English. How strange it seemed to be able to read that sign in a land that felt so foreign!

DESTINATION: SITKA, ALASKA

I had decided to do an affiliation in Alaska about two years before, when my occupational therapy program at the University of Washington received a rural pediatric training grant with a training site in Sitka. A few months in Alaska had sounded adventurous to me. It had also sounded like an opportunity to explore the profession within the context of other cultures. Indeed, one of the reasons that I chose to be an occupational therapist was for the opportunity to work in different places and with different peoples. I felt that my training in Alaska would provide new cultural experiences. I was right; both the white and Native American (Tlingit Indian) populations offered glimpses into cultures different than those I have experienced before.

I found that many people still held frontier values (values that seemed to esteem self-reliance, freedom, and surviving, taming, and exploring new lands). Some people led subsistence lifestyles, hunting, fishing, and/or gathering for the majority of their food. The region was bountiful; the herring came by the millions in March to spawn, halibut and salmon were plentiful, and the land was well populated with deer. One could also harvest herring roe (eggs), seaweed, wild berries (salmonberries, blackberries, huckleberries, cranberries . . .). Hunting, fishing, and gathering were not always safe activities, however. The seas were always cold and unpredictable; storms frequently blew in and out without warning, and the land was heavily populated with brown (grizzly) bears. Whether living a subsistence lifestyle or not, most people lived day to day, more aware of and affected by the wildlife, the land, the weather, and the seasons than my urban counterparts had in Seattle.

Sitka turned out to be an idyllic town. Located on the Western edge of Baranof Island, and facing the Pacific Ocean, Sitka was backed by a cloak of evergreens (part of the 16.9 million acre Tongass Forest). At three thousand feet the trees gave way to snow capped rocky peaks. No roads entered the forest (although there were fourteen miles of road in and around town), so Sitka was as isolated as most other towns and villages in Alaska. The only access to Sitka was via boat or airplane. The town itself was pretty, with a mix of historic Russian buildings and modern buildings, and two college campuses. There were views of the water and mountains from almost anywhere in town. Sitka felt like a modern shelter in the middle of a wilderness that from the ferry had seemed endless and impenetrable. The weather was mild compared with the rest of the state; fifty inches of snow and fifty inches of rain per year. The town's economy was based on trades such as fishing and pulp mill work, and on services such as teaching and health care. The population was eight thousand, making Sitka the fifth largest town in the state (Roppell, 1982).

OCCUPATIONAL THERAPY IN SITKA

My supervisor, Mo McBride, was the sole occupational therapist providing service for all of the schools in Sitka (five public schools, plus several private preschools), and the only occupational therapist in town. In addition, there was no physical therapist working in the schools, so Mo handled all gross motor concerns. This gave me the opportunity to learn and practice the "developmental" model of therapy, having to assess and treat both gross and fine motor functioning. Mo and I also saw any infants who were considered to be high risk for developmental delay. This additional role necessitated a broad knowledge base, and the flexibility to work within both the medical and educational models (because the infants were often in the hospital).

I was Mo's first student, and the first pediatric student in Alaska! The majority of the children receiving occupational therapy services had handicapping conditions such as developmental delay, learning disabilities, and attention deficit disorder. My caseload included children with developmental delay and learning disabilities (several secondary to fetal alcohol effects), attention deficit disorder, hearing impairment, blindness, muscular dystrophy, and Down Syndrome.

As therapists (I was in the position of playing "student" and "therapist" roles at the same time, having passed my occupational therapy boards prior to going to Alaska) we performed all of the duties of typical school therapists "in the lower 48." We assessed children that were referred by teachers or parents who had concerns about a child's perceptual and/or motor skills. We provided direct service for children that qualified with a "handicapping condition" land who were having difficulty functioning in their classroom environment.

We incorporated several treatment frames of reference in direct intervention with the children. With younger children our approach combined the sensory-motor and the developmental frames of references. In the OT-led physical education class for the special needs pre-schoolers we often incorporated obstacle courses into the gym time, using tunnels and climbers. We also frequently used scooter boards on ramps and in group games. We constantly worked on developing beginning group game concepts such as taking turns, interacting in a structured way with peers, and following two- and three-step verbal directions. With older children we tended to use only the developmental approach, often working on perceptual-fine motor skills that they needed to improve handwriting or other classroom related skills. I worked a forty-hour week, although I often spent extra hours at work.

The equipment and treatment spaces that we used were similar to what I have experienced in schools in Washington, although because there was no center based program in the district there were no "therapy" rooms. Mo's office, which she shared with one of the speech therapists in the district, was the only designated occupational therapy space in the district. It was located in the new elementary school, and it was fairly large, with three desks plus a large treatment space that Mo had set up with a computer and a table and chairs. For any one-to-one gross motor work with children we scheduled time in the gym of that child's school. For one-to-one perceptual-fine motor work we usually scheduled time in an empty classroom or office.

One of the things that I appreciated most, professionally, in Sitka, was the practice of integrating children with handicapping conditions into schools and/or classrooms with typically developing children of the same age. There was no center for children with special needs in Sitka, and as a result children with special needs tended to be in the environment that was the "least restrictive" for them. In addition, there was some administrative support for integrating these kids to the fullest degree, by bringing the special services to them in a regular educational program. I was able to reinforce the concept of integration for myself by going to a conference in Anchorage that spoke a great deal to that topic. It was exciting and challenging for me to return to Sitka and try to put that concept of complete integration into practice.

A UNIQUE CULTURE
AND A UNIQUE PROFESSIONAL LIFE

The biggest differences, however, that I now recognize between practice in the "lower 48" and in Alaska came not with assessment tools, treatment practices, or equipment that we used, but with the unique socio-economic situation of Alaska, and with day to day interactions with students, parents, and teachers.

I found that like people everywhere, the parents in Sitka wanted the best for their children. But the "best" was sometimes different than what I had experienced in Seattle. In Alaska a full, formal education did not necessarily lead to a higher quality of life. In fact, teenagers and even children could go out on fishing boats with their parents and earn good money, and often the school calendar interfered with the fishing seasons. This meant that some children were not in school for a full year, or that they were taught at home. For children in these situations who were eligible for special services, it took some effort to first identify them and to then develop a program that fit with their individual needs.

Even in the schools, fishing and sea life played significant roles. Curricula were adapted to teach about the sea's role as a vital resource. Starting in kindergarten all of the children in Sitka learned to swim as part of their school program. In the elementary schools Seaweek was a week-long celebration of the sea and what it brought to life in Sitka. In high school, classes such as marine biology were offered. As part of one of my student's occupational therapy program I accompanied him on a Seaweek fieldtrip to the beach; there we addressed visual-perceptual skills (keeping up with the other kids in finding shells and other "treasure hunt" items on the beach), visual-motor skills (drawing pictures of the totem poles at the park), and gross motor skills (walking and running on the shifting sands).

The pace in Sitka was slower than I had been used to in Seattle. Life did not seem to be ruled by the quick changes and constant deadlines that ruled urban life "down South." Part of this difference was because we were in a rural community. As in small towns anywhere in the United States there was no need to plan ahead — running into friends and co-workers at the post office or at the grocery store was a sure bet. Another part of the difference seemed to be caused by the physical distance from the rest of the United States; the policies and economics of the rest of the country did not feel powerful enough to reach us in Alaska. The influence of the Tlingit culture also added to the difference in pace and lifestyle; their culture places little value on appointments and schedules. Their lives appeared to be lived day by day, and decisions influenced by family needs, the weather, and the season. Thus, I also learned to take things day by day, and to live and work not only by my schedule, but by the weather and by other people's needs.

My first experience with this was when I was scheduled to fly to a remote village about one hundred miles from Sitka to see a three-year-old child who had Down Syndrome. I was traveling with the infant learning teacher, and we were supposed to leave on a Wednesday morning. But a storm rolled in and the trip by small float plane was postponed. We were put on hold until the weather broke. The next morning we were given thirty minutes notice of our flight's departure. During the interim I had to make the time productive, and I had to reschedule the rest of my week accordingly.

Alaska's economy was another unique factor that affected my professional life. Because of high oil revenues Alaska was quite wealthy. In fact, instead of paying state taxes, each resident of the state received an annual dividend from the state's surplus monies! As a result the schools in Alaska were well funded (relative to schools "down South"). Indeed because of the economics of the state, and of Sitka itself, the teachers in Sitka were some of the best paid and most respected people in town. And as a therapist, better funding translated to more support for continuing education, and to somewhat easier access to new playground, therapy, and computer equipment! As an example of this, one of the high schools in Sitka, a school of one-hundred eighty students, had ninety Macintosh personal computers for student use.

The isolation of Sitka was the biggest factor that affected my professional life and development. I sometimes felt apart from the rest of the world — almost trapped in the middle of the wilderness — and I wondered how and what and why the rest of the therapists in the world did whatever it was that they did. I discovered quickly that communication with the rest of the world was vital to my professional growth and to my mental health! I kept in close touch with my advisor from the University of Washington occupational therapy program, Susie Cunningham. I received valuable support from her, and also maintained contact with my familiar occupational therapy world through her. I also countered the professional isolation by continually consulting with Mo, and with the various other professionals in town, such as the speech therapists and teachers. I discovered that this was not only enriching for me, but also for the children's programs, and in addition this communication promoted a solid team approach. Yet another way that I kept in touch with the rest of the world of therapy was by reading journals and other literature. Mo kept a wonderful library of current journals and books, so that was easy for me to do. I also discovered that conferences were more than just informational workshops. At the conference that I attended in Anchorage I realized that networking with other professionals was just as important as getting the information being presented. Telecommunications also played an important role in Alaska — especially when working with people in outlying villages. At times we even had team meetings by teleconferencing.

The isolation in Sitka also served to nurture my ability to problem solve and think independently. I had to trust myself and know my own abilities and limitations. I was often in situations where I was the only person available for the job, and I found that often people wanted or needed answers on the spot. This felt almost frightening, being a "student," and I learned to step back and appraise the situation. I learned that it was alright to not give answers right away. I discovered that it was often more professional to wait and get more information before offering advice or services.

CONCLUSION

Alaska did not turn out to feel like the foreign land that had at first impressed me. By the end of my three and one-half month stay I felt quite at home in the wilderness. In fact, I have had mixed feelings about being back in Seattle. I am still not sure if I prefer to protect myself from people instead of bears, and I certainly miss the beauty and vastness of that great land "up North." I also miss the professional climate; the opportunity to know not only every student receiving therapy in the school district, but every therapist in the state, and at the same time the opportunity to work independently in a climate that supports teamwork and integration. I am able, however, to apply nearly everything that I learned up North here in the "South," because I learned about relating to people and adjusting to other's cultures, and I will carry that with me wherever I work.

REFERENCE

Roppell, P., (Ed.). (1982.) *Sitka and its ocean/island world*. Anchorage: The Alaska Geographical Society.

OF RELATED INTEREST

This column will provide information about professional groups and organizations outside occupational therapy which may be of interest to those wanting information related to the articles in this issue.

The *American Anthropological Association* (AAA) is the largest organization devoted to anthropology in the world and invites as its members anyone with a professional or scholarly interest. The Association has 26 units which represent special interests within the field of anthropology. Some units which might be of particular interest to occupational therapists are: American Ethnological Society, Association for Feminist Anthropology, Council on Anthropology and Education, Society for the Anthropology of Work, Society for Cultural Anthropology, Society for Humanistic Anthropology, Society for Medical Anthropology, Society for Psychological Anthropology and the Society for Urban Anthropology. Most of these units have their own publications and sponsor conferences and workshops related to their areas of interest. For more information about the AAA and these special interest groups, contact: The American Anthropological Association, Membership Department, 1703 New Hampshire Avenue NW, Washington, D.C. 20009.

CONTINUING DISCUSSION ON:
Occupational Therapy Literature Information Services

David Roberts

In a recent issue of this journal (volume 7, no. 1) Ernest (1990) described an information service to some of the journal literature of occupational therapy. This drew attention, if only by implication, to the relatively poor coverage of occupational therapy literature by major information services, including Index Medicus and Excerpta Medica. The extent of the selectivity of coverage of these services seems not to be widely realized (Roberts, 1990a) nor does the fact that the omission of a journal does not necessarily reflect on its quality. (As, for example, stated in the National Library of Medicine's guidelines on journal selection for Index Medicus.) The journal literature of rehabilitation and related areas, including occupational therapy, may be particularly neglected, as some recent studies have shown. For example, Bohannon and Tiberio (1990) compared the coverage by four information services of titles identified by citation patterns of physical therapy journal authors. A study in rehabilitation literature (Bohannon and Roberts 1991) showed similar trends as have two as yet unpublished studies by this author, one a citation analysis and the second based upon identifying titles from serials databases. A recent description of the utility of Index

David Roberts has 15 years experience in Medical Information Service as Index Medicus/Medline indexer and searcher. He is one of the founders of the complementary medicine and allied health database (CATS/AMED). David has recently researched and published on the topic of journal coverage by medical databases, especially in the rehabilitation area. His address is: Medical Information Service, British Library, Boston Spa, Wetnerby, West Yorkshire, LS23 7BQ, United Kingdom.

Medicus for occupational therapists to some extent reinforces this impression, if from a different perspective (Roberts, 1990b).

That supplementary information services for the occupational therapy literature are required therefore seems clear. The service described by Ernest (1990), OTDBASE, attempts to address this question of coverage by including several occupational therapy journals from about 1970 onward. This approach represents an improvement in terms of coverage compared with Index Medicus and Excerpta Medica and may have advantages in other respects as briefly mentioned below. However, a detailed inspection of the journal titles identified in some of the studies referenced above suggests that, in terms of coverage, the approach is limited.

In particular, the British Journal of Occupational Therapy (BJOT) is not included. Occupational therapy has been practiced in Britain for more than 50 years and BJOT, the national journal, was itself established more than 50 years ago. It has been identified as a journal important for occupational therapists in the studies mentioned above though not in two earlier but important studies based upon citation analysis (Johnson & Leising, 1986) (Reed, 1988). The inclusion in OTDBASE of the national journals of Australia and Canada indicates that it is not limited to American journals. The omission of BJOT therefore seems notable.

There is an alternative information service in occupational therapy journal literature, now quite widely used in Britain, though perhaps still relatively unknown in the United States. This is Occupational Therapy Index (OTI) and has been described by Roberts (1988). It has embodied a rather different approach to that of OTDBASE in that, within certain limits, every attempt is made to include all occupational therapy journal literature, including that of relevance appearing in journals of other fields. The limits mentioned are mainly of language (English only), time (1986 onward) and scope, a somewhat difficult matter of definition. The Index appears monthly in hardcopy and typically each issue contains about 100 citations. It is also available as part of a database (known as CATS or AMED) at the British Library and online through the Karolinska Institute in Stockholm, Sweden (Additional online hosts are anticipated during 1991). The whole database, covering citations from 1986 onward, contains a large proportion of material unique to the system and covers the topics: rehabilitation, physical therapy, occupational therapy and complementary (alternative) medicine. In general, abstracts are not included. For further details see Roberts (1988).

The differences between OTDBASE and OTI in terms of scope of coverage and in the time period will be apparent. OTI is considerably wider in scope but more limited in time. It is interesting to note some additional differences with respect to some of the other requirements of information systems by users.

The first of these additional requirements to be mentioned is that of retrieval by subject. The user needs to be able to identify citations on particular topics. This is usually achieved by the assignment of subject headings or descriptors which match the subject content of an article. Subject indexing for information retrieval is a controversial and highly complex matter. A recent extended and authoritative discussion is a monograph by Lancaster (1986). While there is perhaps little consensus in most areas of information science, the experience of online searchers throughout the world for more than a quarter of a century does support the contention that effective retrieval in practice is dependent upon systematic, structured and comprehensive indexing.

Ernest's article gives a list under the heading "OTDBASE Index" which presumably serves as the indexing vocabulary. This list does not correspond to any of the indexing systems used in any of the main medical databases. It seems to lack any coherent structure and, from the information given, to be too general. It may be of interest to contrast this with the approach of OTI. This has been to adopt the Index Medicus vocabulary as a model with the addition of new headings specific to the subject. For example the heading MODEL OF OCCUPATION has been added for the indexing of this important occupational therapy concept. Such an approach has many advantages including compatibility with other databases, relative ease to users who search several databases and more effective retrieval of relevant citations.

The second requirement is that of information—users will want a system to provide as much information as possible. In addition to the basic citation, authors and title, a well-written abstract will often give the reader the clearest indication of the content of an article. The provision of abstracts therefore on OTDBASE may be a considerable advantage from the point of view of the user. The absence of abstracts in OTI is principally due to economic constraints.

Finally, there is the question of availability and awareness of the service. The immediate availability of an information service at the workplace is likely to increase its frequency of use. Availability itself may be influenced by awareness among potential users of the existence of the service. In this, geographic and economic factors may be crucial. In Britain, OTI seems to have been well received and appreciated by occupational therapists in spite of the fact that access has been only to a hardcopy version until very recently. On the other hand awareness of this service in the United States is probably low. Similar consideration will probably affect the utilization of OTDBASE.

It can be concluded that no information service is fully comprehensive and that this is as true of the occupational therapy literature as of any other software. The two information services discussed here will each be of value to occupational therapists. Their strengths and emphases seem to vary so that, to a considerable extent, they may complement each other. This discussion reinforces a point made on many previous occasions that all seeking information should use more than one source or service.

REFERENCES

Bohannon, R.W. and Tiberio, D. (1990). Physiotherapy literature in medical indexes: How comprehensive is index coverage of journals cited frequently by five physiotherapy journals? *Physiotherapy Practice*, 5, 201-205.

Bohannon, R.W. and Roberts, D. (1991). Core journals of rehabilitation: Identification through index analysis. *International Journal of Rehabilitation Research*, *14* (in press).

Ernest, M. (1990). OTDBASE: An occupational therapy literature search service. *Occupational Therapy in Health Care*, 7(1), 127-33.

Johnson, K.S. and Leising, D.J. (1986). The literature of occupational therapy: A citation analysis study. *The American Journal of Occupational Therapy*, *40*, 390-396.

Lancaster, F.W. (1986). *Vocabulary control for information retrieval*. 2nd Ed. Arlington, Va: Information Resources Press.

Reed, K.L. (1988). Occupational therapy articles in serial publications: An analysis of sources. *Bulletin of the Medical Library Association*, *76*, 125-130.

Roberts, D. (1988). A new information service for occupational therapists. *The British Journal of Occupational Therapy*, *51*, 353-354.

Roberts, D. (1990a). Information databases. *The Lancet*, *335*, 917.

Roberts, D. (1990b). Index Medicus and Medline for occupational therapists. Part 1: An overview of coverage and searching methods. *The British Journal of Occupational Therapy*, *53*, 317-20.

An Ernest Response
to Roberts' Comments

Marilyn Ernest-Conibear, MA, OT(C)

Mr. Roberts' comments to "OTDBASE: An Occupational Therapy Literature Search Service" (Ernest, 1990) refer to what he considers to be two important omissions in that article. His first concern was that, although OTDBASE contains extensive and relatively long-term coverage of eight occupational therapy journals published in Canada, the United States, and Australia, the *British Journal of Occupational Therapy* (BJOT) was omitted.

In order to explain that omission, I must give a brief history of the development of OTDBASE. When OTDBASE was developed in 1986, it contained articles and abstracts from only three journals, the *Canadian Journal of Occupational Therapy* (CJOT), the *American Journal of Occupational Therapy* (AJOT), and the *Occupational Therapy Journal of Research* (OTJR). I chose these three because I felt they were the journals which most North American clinicians might have in their departments and which would be most used as references. By 1987, at the request of clinicians, I added *Occupational Therapy in Health Care* (OTHC), *Occupational Therapy in Mental Health* (OTMH), *Physical and Occupational Therapy in Pediatrics* (POTP), and *Physical and Occupational Therapy in Geriatrics* (POTG). In 1989, primarily because of interest expressed by an Australian occupational therapy faculty member and a medical librarian, I added the *Australian Occupational Therapy Journal* (AOTJ).

In 1989, the article of concern was submitted to *Occupational Therapy in Health Care*. Between the time the article was submitted

Marilyn Ernest-Conibear, MA, OT(C) created OTDBASE in 1986. Her address is: 3485 Point Grey Rd, Vancouver, B.C. V6R 1A6.

and the time it was published, I added the *British Journal of Occupational Therapy*, (back to 1984) to the OTDBASE service, again at the request of clinicians.

Mr. Roberts' second point related to the British Library *Occupational Therapy Index* (OTI). He wondered why OTI had not been included in what he felt was an otherwise comprehensive-looking list of Indexing and Abstracting Services found in my article. My list of services was obtained from two sources: (1) the page in each journal indicating all the services in which that journal was indexed or abstracted; and (2) cross-referencing that information with the information about each journal as found in *Ulrich's International Periodical Directory*. Neither source gave any indication that any of the eight journals (or BJOT) was indexed or abstracted in OTI (or, for that matter, in OTDBASE).

So, although I was personally familiar with OTI, it was for the above two reasons I did not include OTI in my list of services and, for obvious reasons, I *did* include OTDBASE. It is apparent to both Mr. Roberts and me that our services (OTI and OTDBASE) are not yet well enough known to be included as indexing/abstracting services in the individual journals, a situation I am sure we both hope will be remedied in the future, not particularly for our benefit, but rather for the benefit of those searching for occupational therapy literature.

I believe a final observation is in order. Occupational therapists are indeed fortunate to have three indexing services dedicated to their literature. The British-based *Occupational Therapy Index* (Roberts, 1988) provides a broadly-based (not only occupational therapy literature, but also other periodical literature of interest to occupational therapists) indexing service. The American Occupational Therapy Association's broad-based library of occupational therapy literature in *OT SOURCE-OT Bibsys* (AOTA, 1989) provides ". . . books, doctoral dissertations, master's theses, SIS newsletters, unpublished research funded by the American Occupational Therapy Foundation (AOTF), and articles from various occupational therapy journals, including the *American Journal of Occupational Therapy* and *Occupational Therapy and Rehabilitation*. The third indexing service, the Canadian-based *OTDBASE* (Ernest, 1990) provides a more narrowly-based *only* occupational therapy journal articles/abstracts search service. Each service fills a different need, and each service complements the other two services. With time at a premium for most clinicians, faculty, and students who wish to know more about what is published in and about their own areas of concern, these three services, I believe, will fill an increasing need both to speed up and broaden the search for existing knowledge relevant to the profession.

REFERENCES

AOTA. (1989). Literature Search Services Available. *OT Week*, Nov. 2, p.2.
Ernest, M. (1990). OTDBASE: An Occupational Therapy Literature Search Service. *Occupational Therapy in Health Care*, 7, 127-133.
Roberts, D. (1988). A New Information Service for Occupational Therapists. *British Journal of Occupational Therapy*, 51, 353-4.

Index

Printed and bound by CPI Group (UK) Ltd, Croydon, CR0 4YY

28/10/2024

01780217-0001